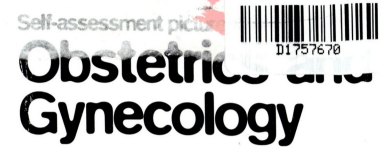

Self-assessment pictures

Obstetrics and
Gynecology

Professor V R Tindall
MD, FRCS, FRCOG
Emeritus Professor of Obstetrics and Gynecology
University of Manchester
England

Roger Baldwin, London
Dr C H Buckley, Manchester
Professor G M Turner, Auckland

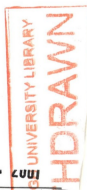

London · Baltimore · Barcelona · Bogotá · Boston · Chicago · London · New York · Singapore · Wiesbaden

Development Editor: **Gina Almond**

Project Manager: **Jane Tozer**

Index: **Nina Boyd**

Design: **Greg Smith**

Cover Design: **Lara Last**

Publisher: **Rebecca Whitehead**

Copyright © 1997 Times Mirror International Publishers Limited

Published in 1997 by Mosby-Wolfe, an imprint of Times Mirror International Publishers Limited

Printed in Italy by Vincenzo Bona s.r.l., Turin.

ISBN 0 7234 2554 X

Contents

Preface

This book is derived from material originally collected for two separate books of self-assessment picture tests and illustrated case histories. Combining examples of both these types of presentations with some multiple choice questions was thought to be more useful for undergraduate and postgraduate medical students as well as for nurses and midwives in training. Both common and less common conditions are covered in all sections.

One could not produce this book without considerable help from colleagues involved in the care of women and in particular those women who allowed their clinical details to be presented. This book is dedicated to them and to those who endeavour to acquire knowledge of the wide range of physiologic and pathologic events which occur in women's lives.

I would particularly like to thank the co-authors, Mr Roger Baldwin, Dr Hilary Buckley and Professor Gillian Turner. The following colleagues who work, or who have worked, in Manchester have also contributed to this book, Dr Connor Collins, Mr Noel Clark, Professor Dian Donai, Dr Paul Donai, Mr Jim Hill, Mr Simon Leeson, Dr Monika Mader, Miss Sarah O'Dwyer, Dr Sylvia Rimmer, Dr Cynthia Stanbridge, Dr David Warrell, Dr Wendy Yates and my secretaries Mrs Eileen Silver and Miss Lynsey Smith. I would also like to thank the following staff of the Publishers, Gina Almond, Lynda Payne, Jennifer Prast, Jane Tozer and Rebecca Whitehead.

Professor V R Tindall
Emeritus Professor of Obstetrics and Gynecology
University of Manchester

Picture Tests

→ 1

It is unusual to take an intravenous urogram (IVU) during pregnancy, so

(a) Why do you think this X-ray film was taken and what is the diagnosis?

(b) What are the common symptoms that this rare group of pregnant women is likely to suffer from?

(c) What is the likely outcome in 60–70% of women with this problem in pregnancy?

(d) What minimally invasive techniques may be used if there is obstruction of the urinary tract?

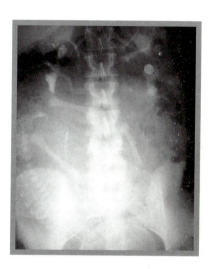

→ 2

(a) If this tumor represented a secondary tumor what do you think the primary diagnosis might be?

(b) How would you establish the diagnosis?

(c) If the report came back that you had completely excised the lesion and there was no evidence of any other lesion would you carry out any further treatment?

(d) Where is another common site for secondary tumors in this condition?

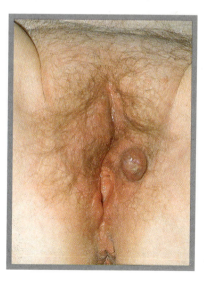

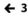

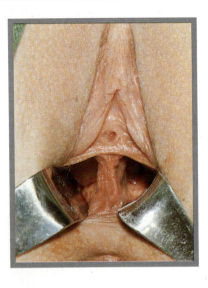

← 3
(a) Is this likely to be an isolated developmental abnormality?
(b) If this lesion was noted in a pregnant patient what difficulties might be encountered?
(c) What gynecological symptoms might this patient have?
(d) What are the risks of dividing the septum?

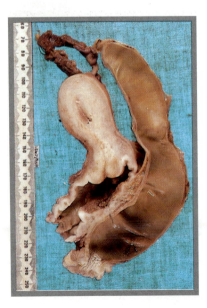

← 4
(a) What is the likely diagnosis in this case?
(b) What operative procedure has been carried out?
(c) What 5-year-cure rate would you give this patient?
(d) What criteria would you require for potential curative surgery in the treatment of this condition?

→ 5
(a) What is the most likely diagnosis?
(b) What are the three most likely enzyme defects?
(c) Is this likely to be a familial condition?
(d) What is the treatment?

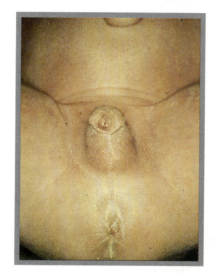

→ 6
(a) This is a uterus with a placenta accreta. Three types of abnormally adherent placentas are described. What are they?
(b) What is placenta accreta commonly associated with?
(c) There is a debate about an aggressive approach or conservative management. What do you understand by these principles?
(d) What are the risks of the conservative approach?

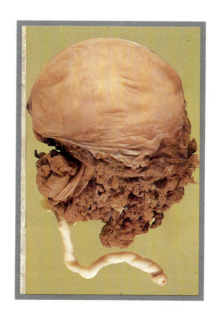

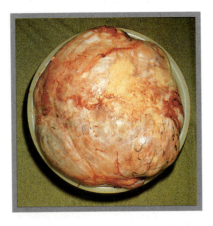

← 7
(a) What is this large solid tumor likely to be?
(b) Is its removal likely to be curative?
(c) If this tumor was ovarian is it likely to be an epithelial or a germ cell tumor?
(d) If this was a benign lesion is it likely to recur?

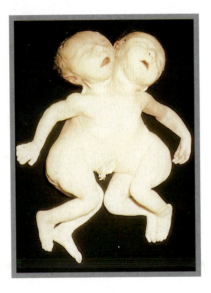

← 8
(a) Is this diagnosis likely to be made antenatally nowadays?
(b) If the diagnosis is made prior to viability what is one option for the parents?
(c) If the pregnancy is allowed to continue what is the management?
(d) Is there a debate about the uterine incision?

→ 9
(a) What is the most likely diagnosis?
(b) What is the treatment?
(c) Is this patient likely to be premenopausal or menopausal?
(d) Why is the infection sometimes difficult to eradicate?

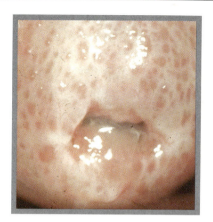

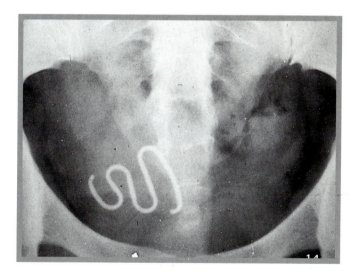

↑ 10
(a) What does this picture show?
(b) Is this likely to be in the uterus or not?
(c) How should it be removed?
(d) What is the incidence of this condition?

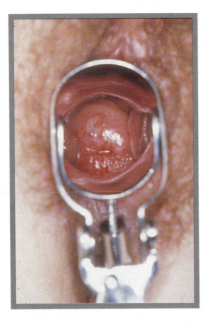

← 11

(a) What is the likely cause of this cervicitis?

(b) In the case of primary infection of the genital tract what proportion of cases will involve the cervix?

(c) Apart from pain at the site of lesions what is the most common symptom when there is cervical involvement? What would you expect cervical cytology in this case to reveal. What would you expect to find?

(d) What is the treatment of this condition?

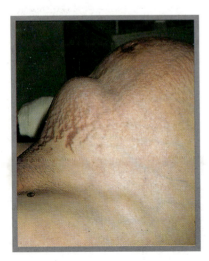

← 12

(a) What is the lower abdominal swelling in this woman in labor?

(b) What do you think was the cause of it?

(c) How would you treat this patient?

(d) Are there likely to be any long-term effects of this?

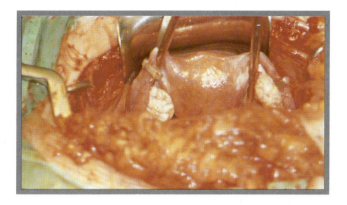

↑ 13
- **(a)** This picture was taken during the course of a hysterectomy operation. What types of clips are applied to the fallopian tubes?
- **(b)** What is a common indication for a hysterectomy after a sterilization operation?
- **(c)** If this patient had requested a reversal of sterilization do you think that it would have been a practical procedure?
- **(d)** Would you remove the clips and part of the tube containing the clips when this patient was having a hysterectomy?

→ 14
- **(a)** What is the diagnosis and how would you treat this?
- **(b)** What do you think was the cause of this?
- **(c)** What investigations might have been carried out before this?
- **(d)** Would it be practical to do a Schauta operation on this patient and would you remove the ovaries?

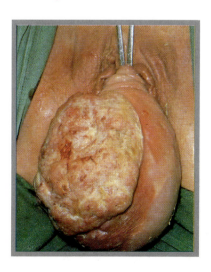

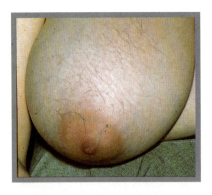

← 15

(a) What are the features of this breast?

(b) What do you think the diagnosis is?

(c) Is any treatment necessary?

(d) What general advice would you give this patient and what are the long-term risks of this condition?

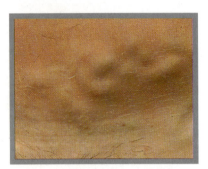

← 16

(a) What does this picture of the lower abdomen show?

(b) What do you think is the cause of this phenomenon?

(c) Is this patient likely to be on any treatment?

(d) If you had to operate on this patient what precautions would you take?

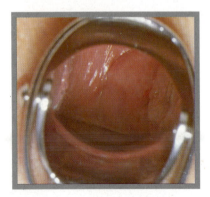

← 17

(a) This picture shows the vaginal vault of a patient who had had a hysterectomy for cervical intraepithelial neoplasia grade 3 (CIN III). What abnormality can you see in the vaginal vault?

(b) How would you make a diagnosis?

(c) If you inspected this with a colposcope what would you expect to see?

(d) What is the long-term risk to this patient?

→ 18
(a) What does this picture show?
(b) Is it likely to be benign or malignant?
(c) How would you treat it?
(d) Is it likely to recur?

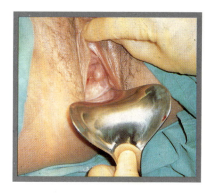

→ 19
(a) What is the diagnosis and what is the plan for treatment after its removal?
(b) What is the incidence of this condition?
(c) What is the likely chromosomal constitution in the majority of cases?
(d) What is the malignant potential of these tumors?

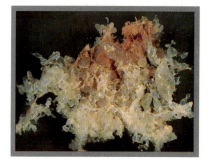

→ 20
(a) Does this young woman have any characteristic stigmata?
(b) What do you think is the likely chromosomal pattern of this woman?
(c) What is the principal gynecological symptom?
(d) What would you expect the follicle-stimulating hormone (FSH) and luteinizing hormone (LH) levels to be and what are the ovaries like in this young woman?

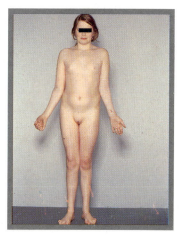

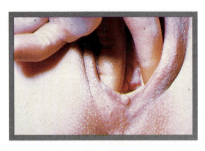

← 21
(a) What does this picture illustrate?
(b) How would you treat it?
(c) Is it likely to recur?
(d) What is the likely etiology?

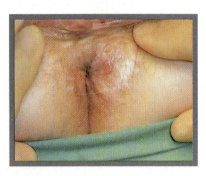

← 22
(a) Would you classify this as an example of vulval dystrophy?
(b) What would be the appropriate treatment?
(c) If the histology report suggested an early carcinoma what would you do?
(d) If the anus and rectum were also involved what would be the appropriate treatment?

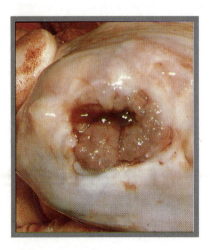

← 23
(a) This is a specimen of a hysterectomy with vaginal cuff retracted. What do you think the diagnosis is?
(b) Do you think that the margin of vaginal epithelium is adequate?
(c) In conjunction with a radical hysterectomy what else might have been carried out?
(d) If the pelvic lymph nodes were involved do you think further treatment would be indicated? What is the prognosis if (i) there is good surgical clearance and no lymph node involvement and (ii) if lymph nodes are involved?

→ 24
(a) What does this cystogram show?
(b) How may this arise?
(c) How may it be treated?
(d) Is this a common condition?

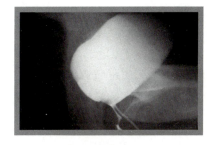

→ 25
(a) What are these bilateral ovarian tumors likely to be?
(b) What is the operative treatment in this particular case?
(c) What is the prognosis of bilateral epithelial tumors?
(d) After surgery what would be the appropriate chemotherapeutic regime?

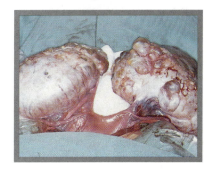

→ 26
(a) What operation is likely to be performed?
(b) What are the current reasons for carrying out a legal abortion in the United Kingdom?
(c) Are there any risks with this procedure? If this was the patient's first pregnancy is there any preparation that you would like to give to the patient before carrying out the operation?
(d) What is the outcome in the majority of cases?

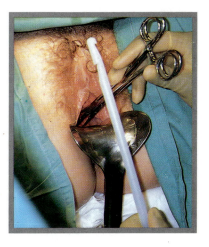

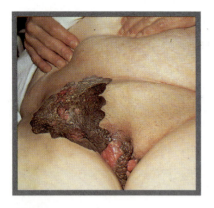

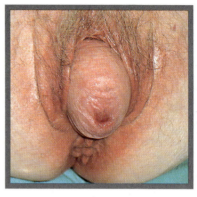

↑ **27**

(a) What is the diagnosis?

(b) What is the appropriate treatment?

(c) In this case the lesion was benign. Would you suggest that the patient is followed up?

(d) Do you think that it would be necessary to carry out a skin graft for this patient?

↑ **28**

(a) What is the degree of prolapse in this case?

(b) What is the treatment? Are there any contraindications to this form of therapy?

(c) What is a recognized sequela of operative treatment?

(d) What advice would you give to the patient regarding postoperative management?

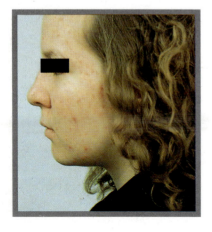

← **29**

(a) This young woman attended complaining of infrequent periods and acne with slight hirsutism. What investigations would you carry out?

(b) Would she benefit from the combined estrogen–progestogen pill?

(c) If she had a regular menstrual cycle and acne what is the treatment?

(d) If this occurred around puberty is it likely to improve when she has a normal menstrual cycle?

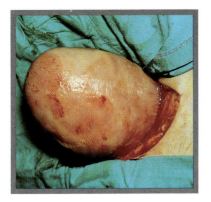

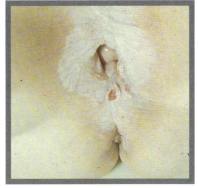

↑ 30
- **(a)** This patient was found to have a single tube and ovary. How do you account for that?
- **(b)** Would you have expected this patient to be fertile?
- **(c)** Would you expect there to be any abnormality of the renal tract?
- **(d)** Why do you think that the uterus is enlarged?

↑ 31
- **(a)** What is the diagnosis?
- **(b)** Is there any other abnormality present?
- **(c)** How would you treat this?
- **(d)** Is there any medical condition that the patient might have?

→ 32
- **(a)** What can you see in this picture?
- **(b)** What could your findings represent?
- **(c)** How would you treat this?
- **(d)** What is the likely prognosis?

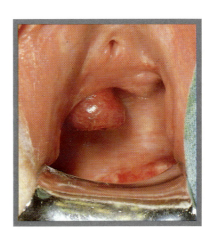

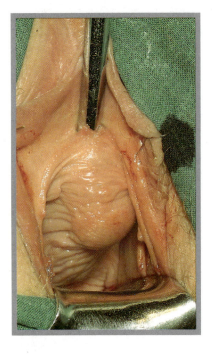

← 33

(a) There is a catheter in the urethra; what else can you see?
(b) How would you treat this?
(c) Do you expect it to be benign or malignant?
(d) Are there any dangers in removing it?

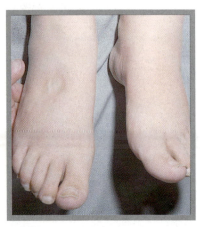

← 34

(a) This woman has pitting edema. What are the likely causes?
(b) If the patient was pregnant what other observations would you make?
(c) If she was a gynecological patient with lymphedema how would you treat it?
(d) Lymphedema can be a persistent problem, particularly following radical surgery and pelvic wall lymphadenectomy. What other gynecological condition may give rise to lymphedema?

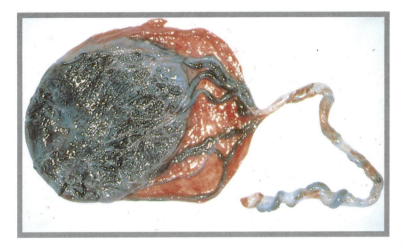

↑ **35**
(a) What is this?
(b) What condition might it be associated with?
(c) Does the placenta look complete?
(d) Is this likely to be associated with retained placenta or with postpartum hemorrhage?

→ **36**
(a) This is an unusual type of ectopic pregnancy, which may be primary or secondary. What are the essential differences between the two types?
(b) This condition is more common in a certain group of women. Which group?
(c) What are the essential criteria for the diagnosis of this condition?
(d) What is the usual outcome?

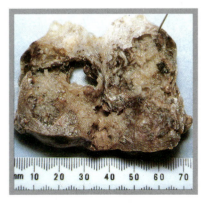

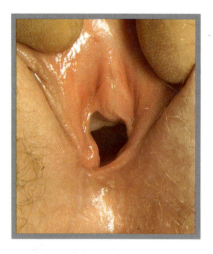

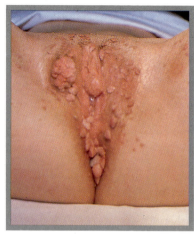

↑ **37**

(a) This woman complained of dyspareunia 6 months after a vaginal delivery. Why do you think this occurred?

(b) What is one operation of choice for treating this woman?

(c) Name an alternative operation.

(d) What is the success rate of these operations?

↑ **38**

(a) What is the diagnosis?

(b) What is their etiology?

(c) Which group of patients is at risk of having them?

(d) What might happen if pregnancy occurs?

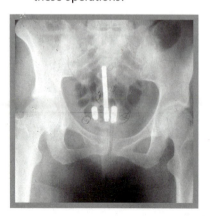

← **39**

(a) What do you think the 'foreign bodies' are in this picture?

(b) What are they likely to contain?

(c) What are they used for?

(d) What is the likely diagnosis?

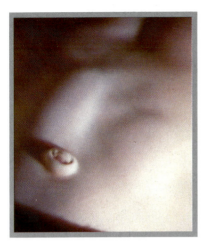

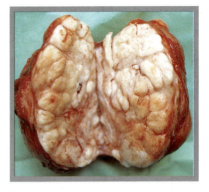

↑ 41
(a) This ovarian tumor was removed from a woman with ascites. What is it likely to be?
(b) What is the common age group for women with this type of tumor?
(c) Are these tumors benign or malignant?
(d) Where else may fluid accumulate?

↑ 40
(a) What is the likely diagnosis?
(b) When does this usually occur?
(c) What are the symptoms?
(d) What is the usual treatment?

→ 42
(a) What is the most likely symptom that this woman would have complained of?
(b) In what age group is she?
(c) What is the most likely diagnosis?
(d) What structures were at risk during the hysterectomy operation? How could the risk be reduced?

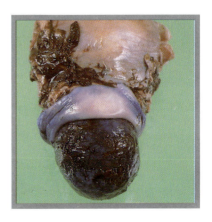

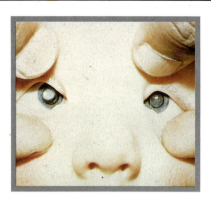

← 43

(a) What do you think is the diagnosis of this child?

(b) What laboratory tests will establish the diagnosis?

(c) What are the neonatal signs and what are the long-term adverse sequelae for the child?

(d) Is maternal screening mandatory?

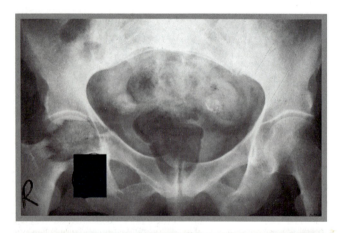

↑ 44

(a) What kind of pelvic infection could these calcified areas reflect?

(b) If this X-ray was taken in a 45-year-old woman, what is the likely medical history?

(c) What is the likely gynecological history?

(d) Is there an association of this pelvic infection with malignancy?

→ 45

(a) What are the two most common conditions that prompt obstetricians to look at the optic fundi?

(b) What is the most likely condition in this picture?

(c) How does this influence the fetal prognosis?

(d) What other organ may be adversely affected in both conditions?

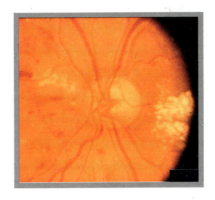

→ 46

(a) What technique is being used in this case?

(b) What conditions are commonly treated with this technique?

(c) Is the treatment usually effective?

(d) What advice would you give to patients after this type of treatment?

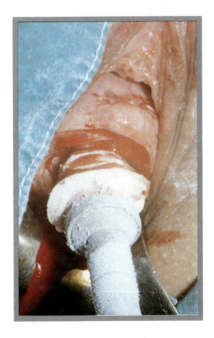

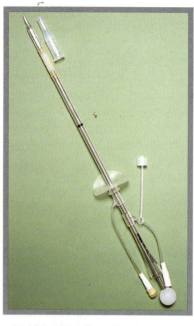

← 47

(a) What are the indications for the use of this equipment?

(b) What are the advantages and disadvantages to the use of this equipment?

(c) Are there any contraindications?

(d) What complications may occur with this equipment?

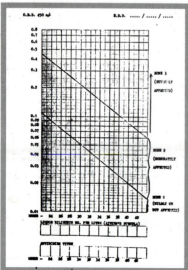

← 48

(a) Why does this chart represent a milestone in obstetrics?

(b) When was it, or a modification of it, introduced into obstetric practice?

(c) What development occurred after the chart was introduced that was related to preventing or avoiding the necessity to use the chart?

(d) What should be the routine for all women having their first pregnancy?

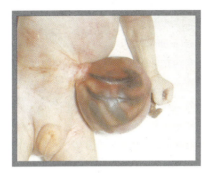

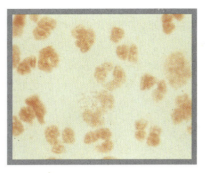

↑ 49
(a) What is the diagnosis?
(b) What tests or investigations might provide a diagnosis antenatally?
(c) What is the most common variety?
(d) What factors influence the prognosis?

↑ 50
(a) What is the likely organism?
(b) Where are the common sites for infection in a symptomless woman?
(c) What is a common concurrent infection?
(d) What is the reason for the organism being relatively insensitive to antibiotics?

→ 51
(a) What does this intravenous pyelogram reveal?
(b) Is it normal?
(c) With what is it associated?
(d) Are there any obstetrical or gynecological risks for this woman?

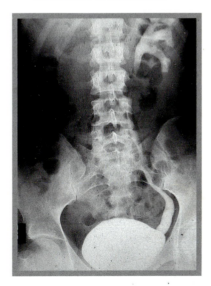

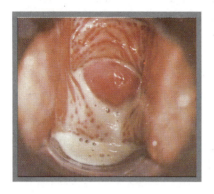

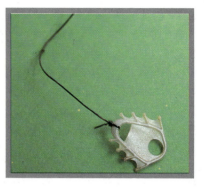

↑ 52
(a) This patient complained of vaginal discharge. What is the probable cause?
(b) What is the causative organism?
(c) How may it be diagnosed?
(d) What is the most appropriate treatment?

↑ 53
(a) This intrauterine contraceptive device (IUCD) has been withdrawn. Why?
(b) How do the current IUCDs work?
(c) Some of the IUCDs are associated with an uncommon bacterium. What is it?
(d) What is the failure rate of IUCDs?

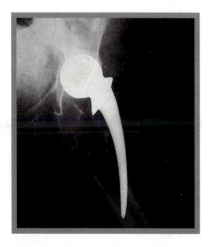

← 54
(a) What is this prosthesis?
(b) What is the likely age group of this woman?
(c) Is it likely that it was a pathological fracture?
(d) Can these fractures be prevented or delayed?

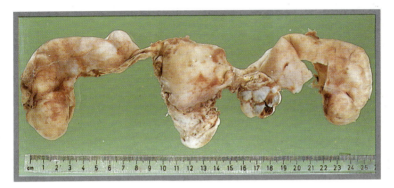

↑ 55
- **(a)** What was the likely indication for the operation?
- **(b)** Does it reflect an acute or chronic condition?
- **(c)** What are the usual causative organisms?
- **(d)** What other organs might be injured during the removal of this specimen?

→ 56
- **(a)** Is this likely to be an infected gland as a consequence of a sexually transmitted disease?
- **(b)** If it is a malignant gland, what are the possible sites?
- **(c)** If an excision biopsy was carried out would any other nodes be removed at the same time?
- **(d)** What is the most likely symptom?

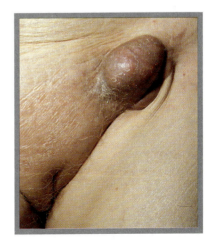

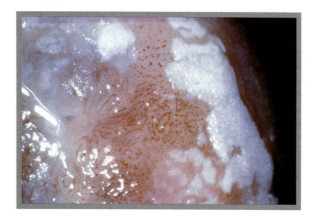

↑ 57
(a) What would you expect a cervical smear to have shown prior to this colposcopy?
(b) How would you describe the findings?
(c) If the white areas reflected a monilial infection would you advise treatment and then reassess by colposcopy?
(d) What would you expect a punch biopsy to show?

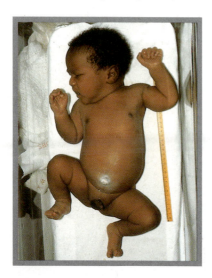

← 58
(a) This child was always 'big for dates'. What is a recognized cause for this?
(b) What test is likely to have been carried out during pregnancy?
(c) What is a recognized hazard during vaginal delivery?
(d) Is this child at greater risk than normal of fetal abnormality if there is a maternal reason for the large baby?

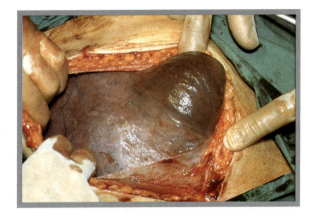

↑ **59**

(a) This is a uterus following a Cesarean section delivery. Is it what you would expect?

(b) What was the likely presentation of the child at delivery?

(c) If delivered vaginally, what is a recognized complication?

(d) Is it likely to have been recognised antenatally?

→ **60**

(a) What is the probable operation to be carried out on this woman?

(b) Why is there evidence of perianal bleeding?

(c) What is the histology likely to reveal?

(d) Will a cure be obtained or is symptomatic relief of symptoms all that can be offered?

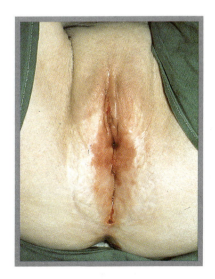

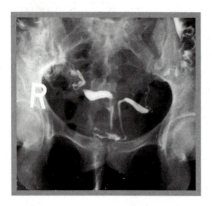

↑ 61
(a) What does this HSG show?
(b) What other abnormalities might you expect?
(c) This woman, when aged 20, suffered dysmenorrhea, which had not been improved by dilatation of the cervices when aged 18. What treatment would you suggest?
(d) What complications may occur in pregnancy?

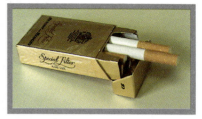

↑ 62
(a) What is the warning given on every packet nowadays?
(b) Why are pregnant women advised against smoking?
(c) Why are cigarettes said to be a factor in cervical cancer?
(d) How would you compare the risk of cigarettes with the risk of taking the oral contraceptive pill?

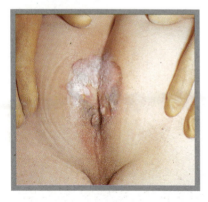

← 63
(a) This diabetic patient had perineal irritation over a 5-year period. She had had recurrent monilial infections that were treated effectively. Are the appearances typical of a monilial vulvitis?
(b) Are the appearances characteristic of vulval warts?
(c) Are the appearances consistent with carcinoma of the vulva?
(d) Which treatment would be the most appropriate: (i) multiple biopsies or (ii) wide excision of the whole abnormal area?

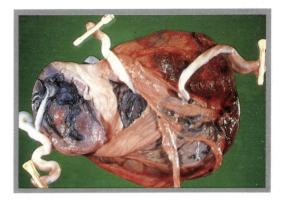

↑ **64**

(a) Is it possible to identify how many fetuses were present?

(b) What is the most common cause of this type of pregnancy nowadays?

(c) What are the recognized antenatal problems associated with multiple pregnancies?

(d) Is there an increased risk of fetal abnormality?

→ **65**

(a) What are the features of this abdomen indicating obstetrical or gynecological procedure(s)?

(b) What do you think the nodule at the umbilicus represents?

(c) If excision biopsy of the nodule confirmed malignancy, what would you do?

(d) What is the prognosis likely to be?

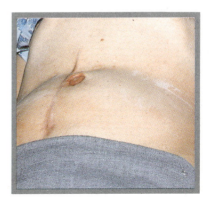

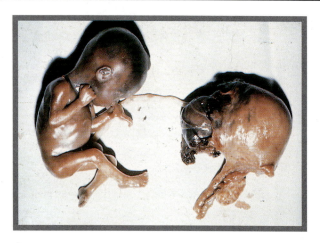

↑ 66
(a) What is your explanation for this ectopic gestation?
(b) At what gestation do you think this rupture occurred?
(c) What advice would you give regarding future pregnancies?
(d) What about the mode of delivery?

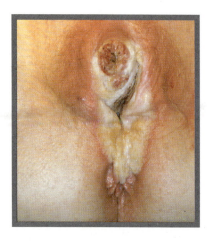

← 67
(a) What is the likely diagnosis?
(b) Where is the likely spread apart from locally?
(c) What is the appropriate treatment?
(d) How much of the urethra can be removed and continence maintained?

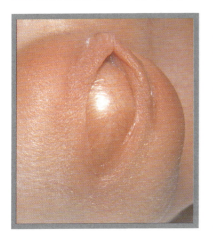

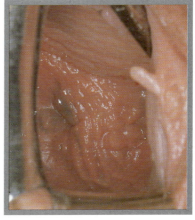

↑ **68**
(a) This is a rare and unusual condition. What is it likely to be?
(b) How would you treat it?
(c) What are the risks of the treatment?
(d) Is this condition usually associated with other abnormalities?

↑ **69**
(a) Is this the normal appearance of the vaginal vault?
(b) What do you think is the likely diagnosis?
(c) How would you treat it?
(d) What are the risks of any operative treatment?

→ **70**
(a) What is the likely diagnosis?
(b) Are they usually bilateral?
(c) When may they occur?
(d) How would you treat them?

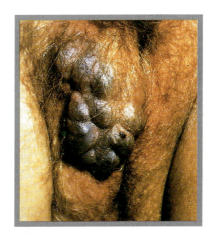

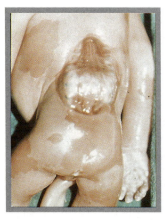

↑ 71
- **(a)** This condition is less common nowadays. Why?
- **(b)** Are there likely to be any other defects?
- **(c)** Are there any prophylactic measures that can prevent these types of abnormalities?
- **(d)** What is the risk of recurrence in future pregnancy?

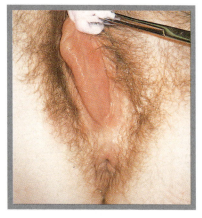

↑ 72
- **(a)** Is this an enlarged edematous labium minus?
- **(b)** What is the treatment?
- **(c)** What is the principal reason for its recurrence?
- **(d)** Would it be appropriate to treat this as a day case?

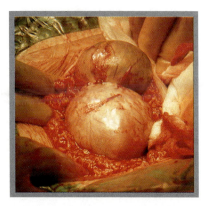

← 73
- **(a)** What structures are visible?
- **(b)** What would you do if the patient was aged 25 years and anxious for a family?
- **(c)** What would you do if the cyst was removed and proved to be an endometriotic cyst?
- **(d)** What would you do if the cyst proved to be a mature teratoma?

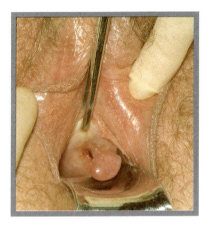

↑ 74

(a) This is a Nabothian follicle. What are they?

(b) How are they formed?

(c) How would this one be treated?

(d) Are they usually single or multiple?

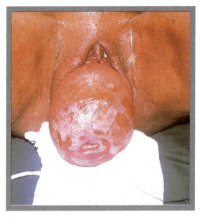

↑ 75

(a) The diagnosis is obvious, but is it long-standing or recent?

(b) What is the operation of choice?

(c) What is a recognized complication after a successful operation?

(d) What treatment would be appropriate if the patient was not fit for anesthesia?

→ 76

(a) What is the diagnosis?

(b) Apart from noticing a lump, what other symptoms may occur?

(c) How should it be treated?

(d) Is it likely to recur?

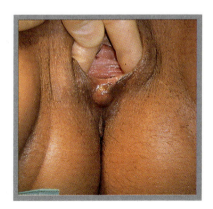

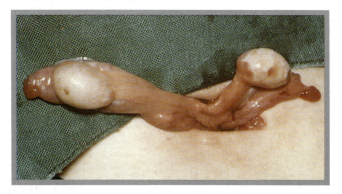

↑ 77

(a) These are gonads of a woman aged 30 years with hirsutism and amenorrhea. What is the likely chromosomal pattern?

(b) Why should the gonads be removed?

(c) What would you expect the histology of the gonads to be?

(d) Would you expect the hirsutism to regress after removal of the gonads?

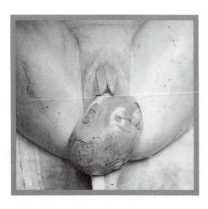

← 78

(a) This is an old slide of a compound presentation. Is it more likely that this baby was dead or alive before labor?

(b) When are compound presentations likely to occur in modern obstetrical practice?

(c) What is another type of compound presentation?

(d) If diagnosed antenatally by ultrasound at 36 weeks, what would you do?

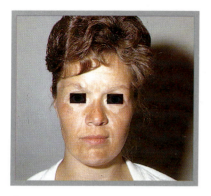

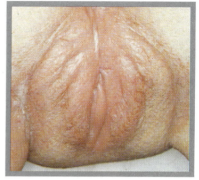

↑ 79
(a) What is the reason for chloasma gravidarum?
(b) Apart from pregnancy, when does it occur?
(c) Where is pigmentation likely to occur in pregnancy?
(d) Does it occur in subsequent pregnancies?

↑ 80
(a) What skin lesion is this?
(b) Does it look as if this is a long-standing condition?
(c) Could it represent a sensitivity phenomenon?
(d) Does this lesion warrant vulval biopsies?

→ 81
(a) This is a colposcopy with saline applied (magnification X 10.) Is this invasive carcinoma or CIN III?
(b) What would you expect the histology of a biopsy to reveal?
(c) Does colposcopy help the diagnosis in this case?
(d) Approximately what proportion of cervical lesions are not squamous?

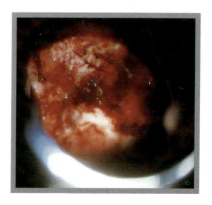

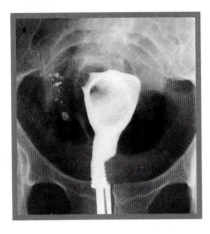

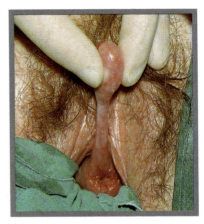

↑ 82
(a) What is the likely diagnosis?
(b) What was the probable clinical reason for this X-ray?
(c) Are there likely to be tumors present and, if so, what is/are their nature?
(d) What complications may occur if pregnancy ensues?

↑ 83
(a) Is this tumor likely to be benign or malignant?
(b) How would you prevent it recurring?
(c) Is there any evidence of uterine prolapse?
(d) What is the presenting complaint likely to be?

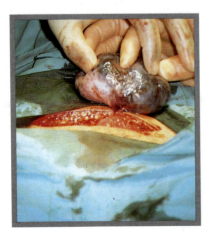

← 84
(a) The presenting symptom was severe pain in a woman aged 25. What is the probable cause?
(b) If, after removal, it was reported to be malignant, what information would you want from the pathologist?
(c) If there were no other abnormal findings in the pelvis and it was reported to be a germ cell tumor, what would be your advice?
(d) What are the possible tumor markers for this type of tumor?

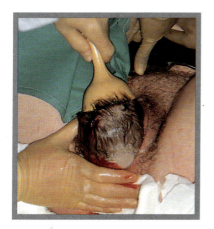

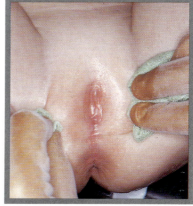

↑ 85

(a) What is the likely reason for the ventouse delivery?

(b) What conditions must be fulfilled before application?

(c) Is an episiotomy obligatory in these types of cases?

(d) What advantage does the ventouse have over forceps?

↑ 86

(a) Why do you think this 3-year-old girl's mother brought her to see a gynecologist?

(b) What local treatment might be beneficial?

(c) Is it a common problem?

(d) Are the labia normal for a girl aged 3 years?

→ 87

(a) What is the likely diagnosis?

(b) Why is an area of the skin marked out?

(c) Do you think you would get primary closure or would a skin graft be more appropriate?

(d) Should the inguinal ligament be divided and the glands removed from the iliac nodes extraperitoneally?

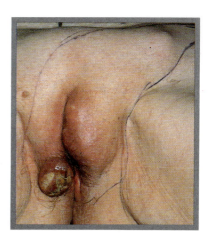

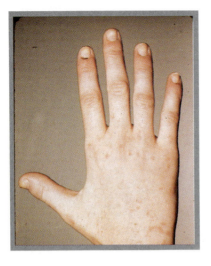

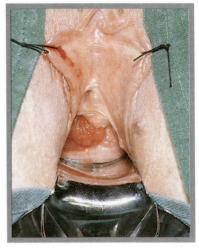

↑ **88**
(a) What is the possible diagnosis?
(b) Are there any risks if this
    woman is pregnant?
(c) Could a diagnosis be made
    from a blood test?
(d) What are the relative risks to
    mother and child if pregnant?

↑ **89**
(a) What is the diagnosis?
(b) What is the likely cause?
(c) What are the chances of cure?
(d) What would be your plan of
    management in a future
    pregnancy?

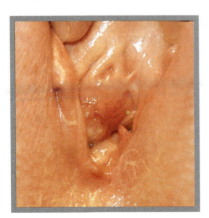

← **90**
(a) What would you expect biopsy
    of the suburethral swelling on
    the right side to show?
(b) Where is it likely to have come
    from?
(c) How would you treat it initially?
(d) What operation might be
    appropriate if it was a recurrent
    tumor with no evidence of
    tumor elsewhere?

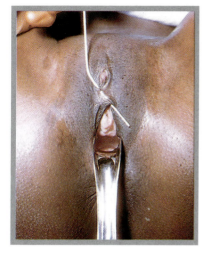

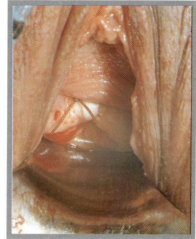

↑ 91

(a) Why do you think the probe can be passed through the fused labia?

(b) Can you name a country where this practice might be carried out?

(c) What are the risks of this practice?

(d) Is it a legal practice?

↑ 92

(a) What operation do you think has been carried out?

(b) What are the recognized complications of this procedure?

(c) What other ways are there of doing this procedure?

(d) What is the usual reason for this operation?

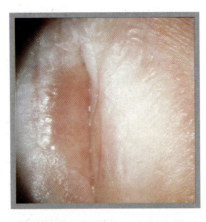

← 93
(a) This is a colposcopy picture (magnification X 10) of the vulval area of a 10-year-old girl. What is the diagnosis?
(b) What is the likely outcome?
(c) In an older woman what treatment may arrest or reverse the condition?
(d) What approximate percentage of cases in the older woman will be complicated by the development of a squamous cell carcinoma?

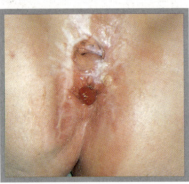

← 94
(a) What operation has this woman probably had previously?
(b) What is the anal lesion?
(c) What operation could you suggest to remove it?
(d) Is there evidence of recurrence?

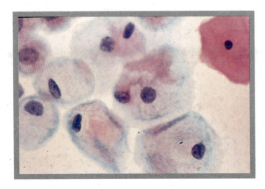

← 95
(a) What does this figure (magnification X 250) show?
(b) What is the significance of these cells?
(c) Where have they come from?
(d) What changes in these cells would concern you?

➔ 96

(a) What structure is being held by the clamps?

(b) What is the lesion on the left ovary?

(c) What are the vessels under the left fallopian tube?

(d) Where is the ureter situated?

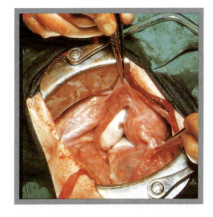

➔ 97

(a) What is the difference between the age incidence of cervical cancer in 1968 and 1979?

(b) Were there more cases in 1968 than in 1979?

(c) What could explain the difference?

(d) Does this graph allow you to assess the number of deaths in the United Kingdom?

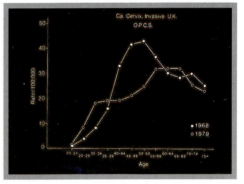

➔ 98

(a) What does this gynecological pelvic ultrasound show?

(b) If this is an ovarian cyst would you consider it to be malignant?

(c) Why?

(d) What is the most likely histological diagnosis?

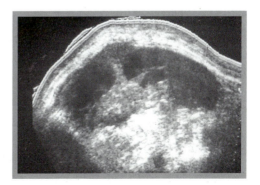

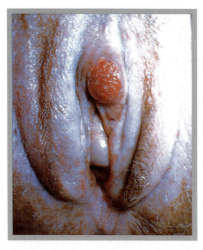

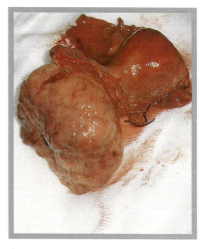

↑ 99

(a) What is the most likely diagnosis?

(b) If it is not malignant what is an alternative diagnosis?

(c) If this is a benign condition what would you do?

(d) Where does this type of benign tumor arise from?

↑ 100

(a) What is this tumor?

(b) If this lesion was 5 cm in diameter rather than 3 cm would it make a difference to the staging?

(c) This lesion was treated by surgery and the ovaries conserved, but would it be sufficient?

(d) What were the likely presenting symptoms?

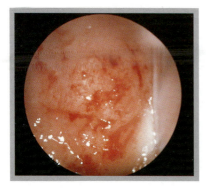

← 101

(a) What does this colposcopy picture (magnification X 16) with saline applied to the posterior lip of the cervix reveal?

(b) What is the likely diagnosis?

(c) If a biopsy confirmed your diagnosis what treatment would you recommend?

(d) Would the treatment proposed be influenced by the age of the woman concerned?

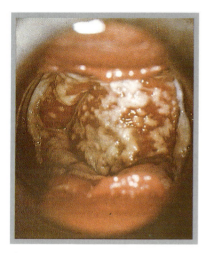

↑ 102
(a) This woman complained of severe vulval irritation. What is the likely diagnosis?
(b) What is the pH of the vaginal surface likely to be?
(c) What are the risk factors for this condition?
(d) What is the treatment?

Triple test report
Maternal details

Age at expected
date of delivery: 30 years
Gestation at date: 16
of sample
Weeks: 3 days (by dates)
Weight: 57.0 kg
Ethnic group: Caucasian

Results

Maternal
serum AFP: 27.4 IU/ml (0.56 MoM)
Oestriol: 2.10 mmol/l (0.56 MoM)
Free
alpha-HCG: 439.1 IU/l (2.19 MoM)
Free
beta-HCG: 24.18 IU/l (1.72 MoM)

↑ 103
(a) What is the significance of this Triple test report regarding Mrs O, a primigravida?
(b) Why?
(c) What is the risk of Down's syndrome at term?
(d) What is the risk of Down's syndrome due to maternal age alone?

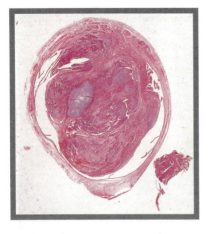

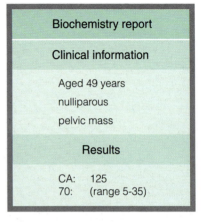

Biochemistry report
Clinical information
Aged 49 years
nulliparous
pelvic mass
Results
CA: 125
70: (range 5-35)

↑ 104

(a) A cross-section of a fallopian tube removed at an emergency laparotomy. What were the likely presenting symptoms?
(b) What is the etiology?
(c) What is the treatment?
(d) What percentage of this group of tumors does this represent?

↑ 105

(a) What is CA 125?
(b) When is it raised?
(c) What action should be taken?
(d) If CA 125 levels are raised postoperatively what does it indicate?

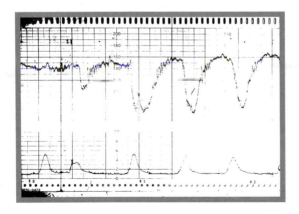

← 106

(a) What is this?
(b) Name three things to be seen.
(c) What action should be taken?
(d) What are the risks of a scalp electrode?

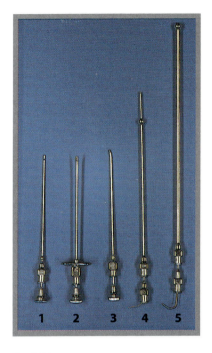

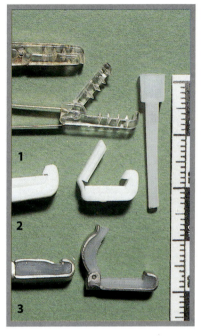

↑ 107

(a) What are the names of these needles?

(b) Before using Nos 1, 2 and 3 what must be done?

(c) What are the limitations for No. 4?

(d) What are the dangers associated with No. 5?

↑ 108

(a) What are these?

(b) What is the failure rate?

(c) Why do they fail?

(d) With what procedure are they usually used?

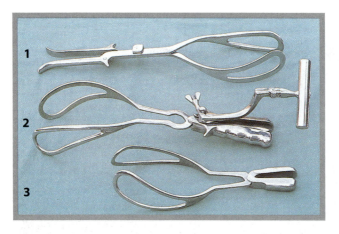

↑ 109
(a) Name these instruments.
(b) Why does the top instrument have a straight shaft and a sliding lock?
(c) What is the danger and advantage of the middle instrument?
(d) Why does the lower instrument have a short handle?

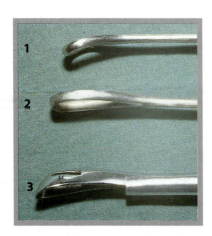

← 110
(a) What are these instruments?
(b) With what hazards are they associated?
(c) With what procedure are they often used?
(d) Why should they not be used alone?

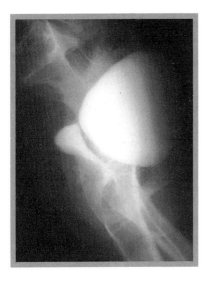

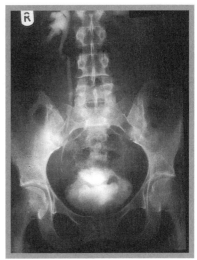

↑ 111, 112
(a) These X-rays were taken 14 days post-hysterectomy. What do they show?
(b) What symptoms would the patient have?
(c) What additional investigations would you undertake?
(d) How would you correct the problem?

→ 113
(a) What is the most likely mode of inheritance?
(b) Could this be an X-linked trait?
(c) Which of the following disorders are associated with this mode of inheritance?
A (i) Huntington's disease
(ii) cystic fibrosis
(iii) testicular feminization
B (iv) neurofibromatosis type 1
(d) What is the risk of A's children being affected and what is the risk to B's children?

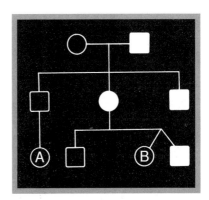

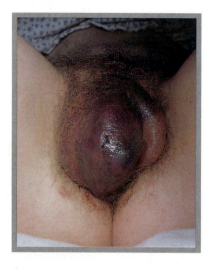

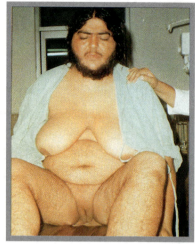

↑ 114

(a) What is the diagnosis?
(b) What sort of accident could cause this type of injury?
(c) How should it be treated?
(d) What are the risks of this type of injury?

↑ 115

This is a gross example of hirsutism.

(a) What are the possible causes?
(b) What investigations would you do to establish the diagnosis?
(c) Is this likely to be physiological or pathological hirsutism?
(d) If nongynecological what are the likely diagnoses?

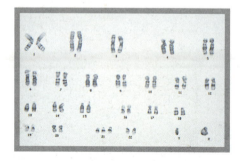

← 116

(a) Is this a normal chromosomal pattern? If not, what does it indicate?
(b) Is the incidence related to maternal age?
(c) If a child is born with this chromosomal pattern is it likely to have any congenital abnormalities?
(d) How could this be diagnosed antenatally?

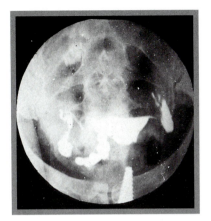

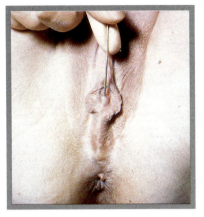

↑ 117

(a) What does this hystero-salpingogram reveal?

(b) What is the etiology?

(c) Apart from infertility what symptoms might this patient have?

(d) Is microsurgery likely to be successful?

↑ 118

(a) What symptoms did this patient have?

(b) What is the treatment?

(c) Could you explain why this occurred?

(d) Is the operation likely to be successful?

→ 119

(a) What is the likely reason for the appearance of the vulva?

(b) What is likely to happen if this patient becomes pregnant?

(c) Is there usually any difficulty with micturition?

(d) Is there any medical justification for this procedure?

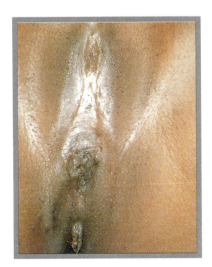

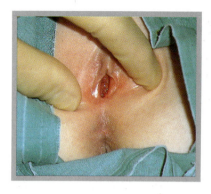

← 120
(a) This patient complained of dysuria and bleeding. What do you think the diagnosis is likely to be?
(b) What age is this patient likely to be?
(c) What is the treatment?
(d) What is the likely histology?

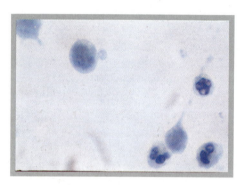

← 121
(a) This is a cervical smear (magnification X 100). What can you identify?
(b) What are its characteristics?
(c) What symptoms does it cause and what is a noticeable feature on examination?
(d) What is an effective drug for its treatment?

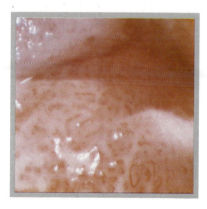

← 122
(a) What does this colposcopy picture reveal?
(b) Does the abnormality extend into the cervical canal?
(c) Are the appearances compatible with 'warty' infection (subclinical papilloma virus infection)?
(d) Approximately what proportion of women with cytological evidence of cervical papilloma virus infection are likely to develop CIN III in 5 years?

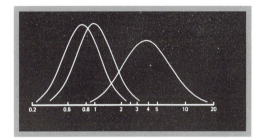

↑ 123
(a) Which of these graphs reflects the normal singleton fetus as far as maternal AFP results are concerned?
(b) Which reflects the likelihood of a spina bifida?
(c) Which reflects the likelihood of Down's syndrome?
(d) What are the chances of the results at given gestations excluding spina bifida and Down's syndrome?

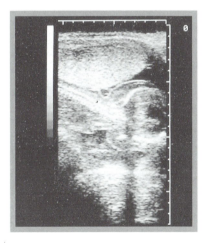

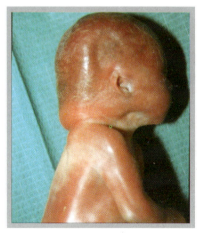

↑ 124, 125
(a) Are there any characteristic features on the ultrasound picture (124) to suggest an abnormal fetus?
(b) Is it acknowledged to be a reliable predictor?
(c) Would the fetus in 125 match the ultrasound picture in 124?
(d) Is there any other characteristic feature visible in 125?

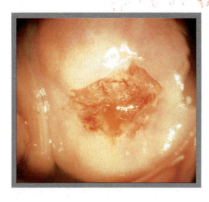

← 126

(a) This woman had abnormal smears for 5 years prior to a cone biopsy. She reattended 3 years later for colposcopy following a further abnormal smear (magnification X 10). Iodine has been applied. What is the significance of the findings?

(b) If her family was complete would you recommend a hysterectomy for CIN III?

(c) Is this lesion laserable?

(d) Is long-term follow-up necessary if a hysterectomy is carried out?

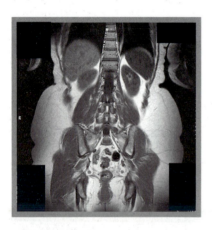

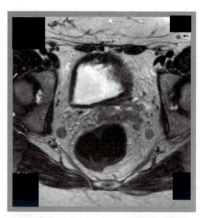

↑ 127, 128

Magnetic resonance imaging (MRI) scans of a woman aged 50 who had a Wertheim's hysterectomy 6 years previously

(a) In the coronal picture (127) what adverse feature can be seen?

(b) Is there any hydronephrosis in 127?

(c) In the axial section (128) what adverse features can be seen?

(d) What are the treatment options?

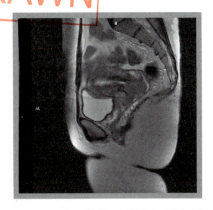

Questions

→ **129–131**

(a) In the sagittal MRI (129) of a woman aged 38 years with postcoital bleeding what can be seen?

(b) In the upper axial MRI (130) what can be seen?

(c) In the lower axial MRI (131) what comment can you make about the parametrium?

(d) What treatment would you recommend?

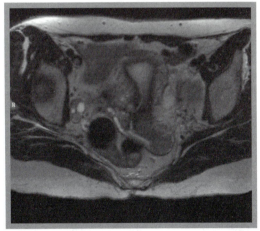

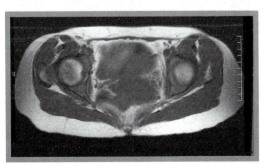

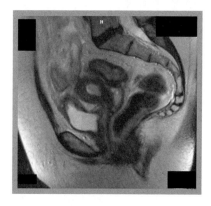 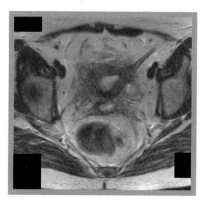

↑ **132, 133**

This patient, aged 53 years, had radiotherapy 2 years previously for carcinoma of the cervix. She returned with pain and a mass.

(a) What does the sagittal MRI (132) reveal?

(b) What does the transverse axial MRI (133) show?

(c) What is the likely diagnosis?

(d) What are the possible treatment options?

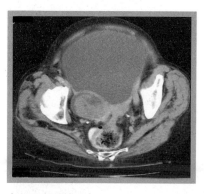 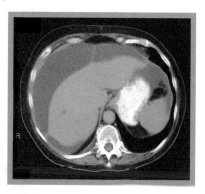

↑ **134, 135**

(a) What does the computerized tomography (CT) scan of the pelvis (134) reveal?

(b) A further scan of the upper abdomen in this patient is shown (135). What does it reveal?

(c) What is the diagnosis?

(d) What is the treatment and likely prognosis?

→ 136

(a) What does this CT scan at the level of the mid-abdomen of a 60-year-old woman reveal?

(b) What do you think the mass in 136 represents?

(c) What operation is required?

(d) Is the operation likely to be palliative or curative?

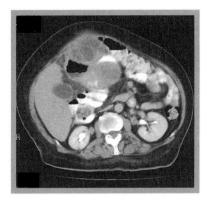

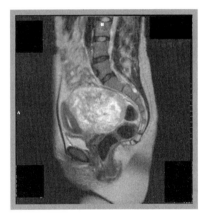

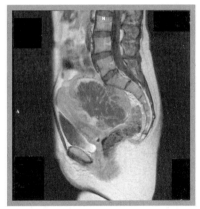

↑→ 137–139

(a) What do the pre- and postcontrast CT scans (137 and 138) reveal?

(b) Where is the mass located in 139?

(c) The primary tumor was relatively uncommon. What is it likely to be, a sarcoma or melanoma?

(d) Is treatment likely to be successful?

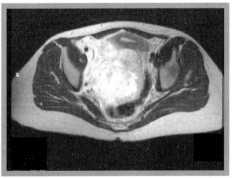

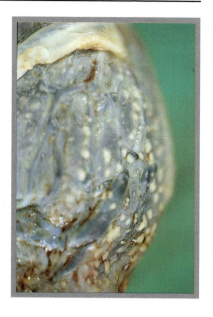

↑→ 140, 141

(a) Do you notice anything unusual with this twin placenta?

(b) 141 reveals a closer view of one of the placentas. What do the white areas represent?

(c) What is their significance?

(d) What is the likely outcome for this fetus?

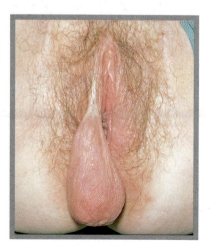

← 142

(a) What is the likely diagnosis?

(b) What does it arise from?

(c) How would you deal with this?

(d) Has it undergone torsion?

→ 143

(a) What does this hysterosalpingogram reveal?

(b) What would be a more appropriate investigation?

(c) If this woman conceived what would be the likely outcome?

(d) Would a myomectomy improve the woman's chance of conception?

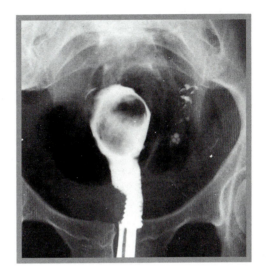

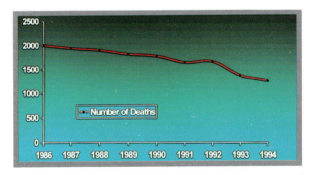

↑ 144

(a) With what gynecological tumor is this likely to be associated?

(b) How do you explain the fall in numbers of deaths from 2000 to 1265?

(c) If the number of deaths from another gynecological cancer was 4000 in 1986, which would it be?

(d) Would that figure show the same rate of fall by 1994?

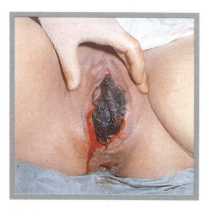

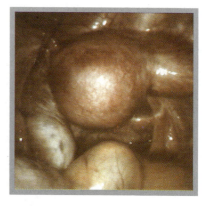

↑ 145

(a) Is this head crowned?

(b) Has the episiotomy been done too early?

(c) What are the advantages and disadvantages of a midline episiotomy?

(d) What approximate proportion of women having their first pregnancy have episiotomies?

↑ 146

(a) This patient complained of recurrent cyclical RIF pain. Can you identify a possible cause in this laparoscopy view of the pelvis?

(b) If this was dealt with by laparoscopy what procedure would be carried out?

(c) What is likely to happen to the right appendage?

(d) Why do you think the operation was done laparoscopically?

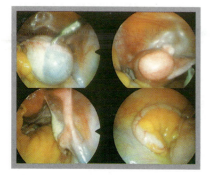

← 147

What do the following laparoscopy findings reveal?

(a) Upper left?

(b) Upper right?

(c) Lower left?

(d) Lower right?

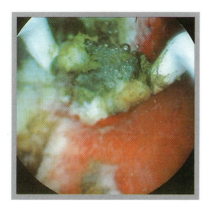

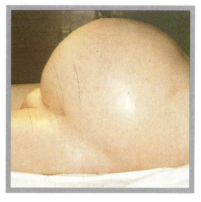

↑ 148

(a) What procedure is being carried out?

(b) What is the principal indication for this operation?

(c) What is the main advantage of this procedure?

(d) What is the main hazard of this operation?

↑ 149

(a) If pregnant would this woman have a multiple pregnancy or polyhydramnios?

(b) If she did have polyhydramnios what would you request the pediatrician to do postpartum?

(c) If pregnant, and the Pfannenstiel incision was from a previous Cesarean section, how would you deliver her?

(d) If this is a gynecological problem is it more likely to be benign or malignant?

→ 150

(a) Are these cells in a cervical smear normal?

(b) What do you think the report would say and what advice given?

(c) What is the essential difference between cervical screening and breast screening?

(d) What are the relative costs of each of these screening programmes?

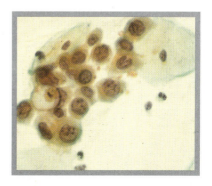

Multiple choice

Which of the following statements are true?

151 Pregnancy aggravates the clinical features associated with

A Eisenmenger's syndrome.
B cutaneous neurofibromatosis.
C von Willebrand's disease.
D SC hemoglobinopathy.
E sarcoidosis.

152 Two years after vaginal hysterectomy a 55-year-old woman develops an enterocele. Which of the following operations would be appropriate and allow preservation of sexual function?

A Le Fort operation.
B Sacrocolpoplexy.
C Sacrospinous fixation.
D Postanal repair.
E Combined abdominoperineal repair.

153 After the vaginal delivery of a first twin

A internal podalic version is an acceptable procedure.
B the ventouse should not be used for the delivery of the second twin with an unengaged head.
C there is no risk of cord prolapse once the presenting part has engaged.
D the second sac of membranes should be ruptured at once.
E the second twin should ideally be delivered within 20 minutes.

154 Ovarian (cystic teratoma) dermoid cysts characteristically

A are associated with Brenner tumors.
B arise principally from endodermal embryonal elements.
C are bilateral in approximately 10–15% of cases.
D are associated with ascites.
E present in the fifth decade of life.

155 The procedure of amniocentesis

A is used to detect Down's syndrome by radioimmunoassay of amniotic fluid.
B has a positive Kleihauer test as a recognized sequel.
C carries an increased risk of orthopedic deformity as a sequel.
D carries a risk of chorioamnionitis in 3–5% of cases.
E can be used to reduce excessive production of amniotic fluid.

156 Which of the following are recognized associations? Primary dysmenorrhea and

A endometriosis.
B a cystic corpus luteum.
C ovulatory cycles.
D relief by the administration of prostaglandin synthetase inhibitors.
E elevation of endometrial prostaglandin F2α concentration.

157 Features of massive central pulmonary embolism include

A a raised jugular venous pressure.
B right ventricular strain in the electrocardiogram.
C sinus tachycardia.
D tachypnea.
E pulmonary vascular congestion on the chest X-ray.

158 Down's syndrome

A is more often due to translocation than to non-disjunction.
B is detectable by examination of the chorionic villi.
C can be prevented by periconceptual vitamin supplementation.
D is associated with a maternal serum alphafetoprotein (AFP) below the 5th centile.
E has an incidence in the United Kingdom of approximately 1:600 live births.

159 Which of the following are recognized causes of postcoital bleeding?

A Intrauterine contraceptive device (IUCD).
B Cyst of Gartner's duct.
C Cervical polyp.
D Postmenopausal vaginitis
E CIN III.

160 Recognized associations with breech presentation after 36 weeks include

A cornual–fundal implantation of the placenta.
B a neural tube defect.
C talipes equinovarus.
D subsequent lowered intelligence quotient (IQ).
E congenital dislocation of the fetal hips.

161 In the evaluation of a 17-year-old patient with primary amenorrhea which of the following investigations are indicated?

A Measurement of serum prolactin levels.
B X-ray of the pituitary fossa.
C Pelvic ultrasound examination.
D Measurement of serum gonadotrophins.
E Estimation of urinary beta-human chorionic gonadotrophin.

162 During labor, following one previous Cesarean section

A uterine rupture characteristically occurs at the time of instrumental delivery.
B the incidence of rupture of a 'classical' scar is approximately 20%.
C fetal heart rate abnormalities indicate the possibility of scar dehiscence.
D epidural analgesia is contraindicated.
E the second stage should not exceed 30 minutes.

163 A 35-year-old mother of six requests sterilization. She weighs 91 kg (200 lb) and has an asymptomatic second-degree uterovaginal prolapse. A cervical smear and colposcopic biopsy shows CIN III. Appropriate methods of management include

A vaginal hysterectomy and repair.
B regular cytological follow-up, regardless of whether the cervix is removed.
C urgent cone biopsy.
D low-dose pelvic irradiation.
E local ablative treatment of the cervix.

164 At 42 weeks' gestational age or more

A the most common cause of perinatal death is trauma.
B there is a substantial fall in the fetal hemoglobin level.
C there is a significant preponderance of female infants.
D there is a centre of ossification in the cuboid bone.
E oligohydramnios is a recognized feature.

165 In precocious puberty

A the onset of menstruation will differentiate between true and pseudo precocity.
B there is a recognized association with hyperthyroidism in childhood.
C an organic cause is more likely to be identified in boys than in girls.
D epilepsy is a recognized association.
E granulosa cell tumor is a recognized cause.

166 For a pregnant woman over the age of 35 years there is an increase in the

A frequency of fetal neural tube defects.
B frequency of multiple pregnancy.
C incidence of pregnancy prolonged beyond 40 weeks.
D incidence of maternal hypertension.
E incidence of maternal hyperthyroidism.

167 Adrenal tumors causing hirsutism in women are associated with

A raised levels of adrenocorticotrophic hormone (ACTH).
B cortisol suppression by dexamethasone.
C absence of diurnal cortisol variation.
D raised serum 17-alpha-hydroxyprogesterone levels.
E hyperglycemia.

168 Factors associated with the spontaneous onset of premature labor include

A hydrocephalus.
B oligohydramnios.
C intrauterine growth retardation.
D bicornuate uterus.
E untreated maternal syphilis.

169 In a woman with inappropriate lactation and secondary amenorrhea

A treatment with danazol would be appropriate.
B an increased plasma progesterone concentration would be expected.
C bitemporal hemianopia on perimetry would be expected in about 25% of patients.
D the administration of methyldopa is a recognized cause.
E anorexia nervosa is a recognized association.

170 Which of the following congenital anomalies can be diagnosed by ultrasound imaging at 18 weeks' gestation?

A Congenital dislocation of the hip.
B Beta-thalassemia.
C Spina bifida occulta.
D Congenital adrenal hyperplasia.
E Phocomelia.

171 In treating ovarian cancer, cisplatin

A is the treatment of choice for choriocarcinoma.
B is ototoxic.
C is effective when given orally.
D usually causes alopecia.
E seldom produces severe myelosuppression.

172 Which of the following statements concerning the bony pelvis are correct?

A The sacrosciatic notch is significantly wider in an android pelvis.
B In the anthropoid type of female pelvis, the anteroposterior diameter of the inlet is significantly greater than the transverse.
C A straight sacrum is associated with a narrow subpubic angle.
D The angle of inclination of the pelvic brim is greater in the negroid than in Caucasian women.
E The female pelvis is characteristically shallower than the male pelvis.

173 Procedures of value in the diagnosis of gonorrhea in women include

A the naked eye examination of the vaginal discharge.
B a complement fixation test.
C the examination of the male partner.
D culture of a cervical swab.
E culture of a swab from the anal canal.

174 A previously normotensive primigravida develops a blood pressure of 160/100 mmHg and 4 g of proteinuria each 24 hours for the preceding 7 days. The following features would be expected

A a lowered level of fibrin degradation products (FDP).
B a creatinine clearance of 120–150 ml per minute.
C hyperreflexia.
D loss of diurnal variation in blood pressure.
E papilledema.

175 Shoulder girdle dystocia

A is heralded by head retraction on to the vulva and perineum.
B is to be expected in 20% of women with babies weighing more than 4 kg.
C may cause Klumpke's paralysis.
D is managed by rotating the shoulders into an oblique diameter of the pelvis.
E is associated with a 30% incidence of long-term neurological problems.

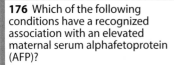

176 Which of the following conditions have a recognized association with an elevated maternal serum alphafetoprotein (AFP)?

A Retroplacental hemorrhage.
B Closed spina bifida.
C Fetal gastroschisis.
D Fetal cystic fibrosis.
E Congenital adrenal hyperplasia.

177 There are recognized associations between Gram-negative septicemia and

A leucopenia.
B clinical response to metronidazole.
C abscess formation.
D septic thrombophlebitis.
E endocarditis.

178 Diseases that have a recognized association between maternal infection during pregnancy and fetal congenital anomalies include

A mumps.
B brucellosis.
C malaria.
D genital herpes simplex virus type II.
E hepatitis B.

179 The risk of thromboembolism after surgical operations is reduced

A in patients with blood group O compared with those of blood group A.
B in thin compared with fat people.
C in nonsmokers compared with smokers.
D by preoperative administration of subcutaneous heparin.
E by the intravenous infusion of Hartmann's solution during operation.

180 Which of the following statements regarding occipitoposterior positions are true?

A Between 10 and 20% of all cephalic presentations are occipitoposterior in early labor.
B In multiparous womens, it is the most common cause of a high head at term.
C Labor is associated with early spontaneous rupture of the membranes.
D An anthropoid pelvis is a recognized predisposing factor.
E The presenting diameter is likely to be the occipitofrontal.

181 In a 35-year-old woman, serum gonadotrophin concentrations are raised

A in Cushing's syndrome.
B with cystadenocarcinoma of the ovary.
C with congenital absence of the ovaries.
D in the androgen insensitivity syndrome.
E with an estrogen-secreting tumor.

182 In maternal thyrotoxicosis complicating pregnancy or the puerperium

A subtotal thyroidectomy is acceptable treatment in the second trimester.
B the condition is best treated by giving a 'blocking' dose of carbimazole together with a normal replacement dose of thyroxine.
C all medication should be withdrawn no later than 6 weeks before delivery.
D neonatal hyperthyroidism does not occur if the mother has been euthyroid.
E the dosage of antithyroid drugs required can be accurately monitored by serial estimation of serum total thyroxine concentration.

183 Which of the following genital anomalies have a recognized association with the conditions listed?

A Inguinal hernia: congenital adrenal hyperplasia.
B Imperforate hymen: Turner's syndrome.
C Persistent cloaca: congenital adrenal hyperplasia.
D Varicocele: Klinefelter's syndrome.
E Hypospadias: androgen insensitivity (testicular feminization syndrome).

184 Recognized associations of the polycystic ovarian syndrome (POS) include

A carcinoma of the breast.
B anorexia nervosa.
C short stature.
D endometrial carcinoma.
E galactorrhea.

185 Which of the following conditions are characteristically associated with oligohydramnios?

A Talipes equinovarus.
B Hemangioma of the placenta.
C Fetal polycystic kidneys.
D Fetal imperforate anus.
E Fetal renal agenesis.

186 A cervical smear can identify the presence of

A *Trichomonas vaginalis.*
B *Chlamydia trachomatis.*
C *Neisseria gonorrhea.*
D actinomycosis-like organisms.
E cytomegalovirus.

187 Prolonged first stage of labor has a recognized association with

A mentoposterior position of a face presentation.
B a breech presentation.
C epidural analgesia.
D a bicornuate uterus.
E maternal dehydration.

188 Conditions that are recognized to predispose to the development of carcinoma of the endometrium include

A previous radiation-induced menopause.
B adrenal hyperplasia.
C hilar cell tumor.
D maturity-onset diabetes mellitus.
E uterine fibroids.

189 Causes of cystic swellings within the female breast include

A fibroadenosis.
B duct carcinoma.
C degeneration within a colloid carcinoma.
D disgerminoma of the ovary.
E long-term use of the combined oral contraceptive.

190 Borderline epithelial tumors of the ovary are characterized by

A multilayering (stratification) of the epithelial cells.
B detachment of cellular clusters from their sites of origin.
C increased mitotic activity.
D stromal invasion.
E nuclear abnormalities.

191 Cytotoxic therapy is the recommended therapy for

A borderline epithelial tumors of the ovary.
B FIGO Stage 1a epithelial carcinoma of the ovary.
C FIGO Stage 1c epithelial carcinoma of the ovary.
D FIGO Stage IV epithelial carcinoma of the ovary.
E stromal endometriosis of the ovary.

192 Conditions affecting the gastrointestinal tract that may also affect the vulva include

A infection with *Oxyuris vermicularis.*
B Crohn's disease.
C ulcerative colitis.
D diverticular disease.
E amebiasis.

193 Which of the following statements concerning rubella are true?

A Maternal infection occurring in the second trimester is followed by the neonatal rubella syndrome in less than 1% of cases.
B The rubella hemagglutination inhibition test becomes positive within 4 days of the infection.
C Viremia precedes the rash.
D Treatment with immunoglobulin reduces the risk of congenital abnormality.
E Conjunctivitis in the neonate is a characteristic feature.

194 Recognized associations with pelvic endometriosis include

A vaginal adenosis.
B uterine fibroids.
C prolonged use of the IUCD.
D hematometra.
E dyschezia.

195 Disseminated intravascular coagulation (DIC) has a recognized association with

A placental abruption.
B multiple pregnancy.
C septic abortion.
D iron-deficiency anemia.
E prolonged bed rest.

196 Which of the following statements concerning trophoblastic disease are true?

A Choriocarcinoma may be accompanied by clinical evidence of thyrotoxicosis.
B Less than 2% develop into choriocarcinoma.
C There is a significant increase in incidence beyond the age of 40 years.
D The prognosis is influenced by the patient's ABO blood group.
E The karyotype is characteristically 46XX.

197 Recognized etiological factors in spontaneous first trimester abortion include

A cervical incompetence.
B celiac disease.
C infection with *Listeria monocytogenes.*
D lack of antipaternal cytotoxic antibodies.
E a deficiency of the beta-subunit of HCG.

198 Which of the following statements regarding the menarche are true?

A Anovulatory cycles are usual for 6–12 months after the onset of the menarche.
B The average time interval from breast budding to menarche is about 2 years.
C The mean age is 10–12 years in girls in America and the United Kingdom.
D The maximal growth spurt occurs after the menarche.
E Pubic hair growth develops after the menarche.

199 Which of the following statements concerning the fallopian tubes are true?

A Torsion after tubal ligation is usually of the distal end.
B Gonococcal infection typically produces a terminal endosalpingitis.
C Carcinoma constitutes approximately 5% of genital tract cancers.
D Pyosalpinx is a common sequel to postabortion infection.
E They are the most common site for genital tuberculosis.

200 With regard to asymptomatic vaginal adenosis, it

A does not require any specific therapy.
B proceeds to carcinoma in less than 10% of cases.
C has a diploid chromosomal pattern.
D occurs only in patients with prenatal exposure to diethylstilbestrol.
E is a recognized complication of herpes simplex virus type II infection.

201 In pregnancy, maternal heroin addiction

A causes an increase in the incidence of low birthweight babies.
B is associated with an increased stillbirth rate if treated by maternal maintenance with methadone.
C leads to a greater incidence of prolonged pregnancy.
D is associated with an increased incidence of meconium staining of the liquor.
E is associated with a greater perinatal mortality rate when treated by maternal detoxification.

202 In pregnant epileptic patients taking phenytoin

A the reduction in plasma drug concentration is mainly due to increased liver metabolism.

B increased protein binding of the drug occurs.

C there is no increase in the convulsion rate if plasma drug levels are maintained in the therapeutic range.

D breastfeeding should be discouraged.

E the neonate requires vitamin K supplements.

204 A young woman miscarries at 14 weeks' gestation and becomes very unwell with a high fever. In looking for a cause the following factors might be of relevance

A that in the past she has suffered from recurrent vulval herpes.

B that she has just acquired a young kitten as a pet.

C that she has recently eaten soft cheese.

D that she lives on a sheep farm.

E that the results of routine serological screening tests for syphilis were VDRL positive, TPHA negative.

203 Conservative management of ectopic pregnancy by intratubal injection of methotrexate

A is contraindicated in the presence of tubal rupture.

B should be limited to cases with a tubal diameter of 3–4 cm.

C is particularly effective when ultrasound examination demonstrates fetal cardiac activity.

D should be followed by serial measurement of serum progesterone until values fall to the nonpregnant range.

E is safe provided that citrovorum factor is administered concurrently.

205 Between 80 and 90% of couples attempting to conceive are successful after 1 year. Which of the following statements are true?

A Tubal damage accounts for about 14% of all causes of infertility.

B Resources currently devoted to tubal surgery for severe disease could be more efficiently used if reallocated to assisted conception techniques.

C Reversal of female sterilization is not effective.

D Diagnosis of tubal damage is best made by laparoscopy alone.

E The ectopic pregnancy rate following surgery for distal tubal occlusion is about 15–25%.

206 In cases of twin–twin transfusion syndrome

A placentation is often dichorionic.
B there is a high perinatal mortality rate when the diagnosis is made before 28 weeks' gestation.
C characteristic umbilical artery Doppler waveforms may be observed.
D fetal hydrops in one twin may resolve following the intrauterine death of the co-twin.
E intrauterine death of one twin may be associated with significant neonatal handicap in the surviving twin.

207 Which of the following statements regarding abnormal vaginal bleeding are true?

A Less than 1% of endometrial adenocarcinomas occur in women under 35 years.
B Approximately 6% of endometrial adenocarcinomas occur in women under 45 years.
C Dilatation and curettage alone will miss 10% of endometrial pathology.
D Dilatation and curettage has been shown to have a greater therapeutic effect than previously thought.
E Endometrial sampling not only avoids general anesthesia but is as accurate as outpatient hysteroscopy.

208 Which of the following abnormalities detected in an 18–20-week ultrasound scan may be associated with trisomy 21 in the fetus?

A Nuchal fold thickening greater than 6 mm.
B Dilatation of the renal pelvis.
C Gastroschisis.
D Banana-shaped cerebellum.
E Femur length shorter than expected for gestational age.

209 In anorexia nervosa, which of the following statements are correct?

A The onset is between the age of 30 and 40 years.
B The weight is 25% below normal for age and height.
C Diarrhea is a common symptom.
D There are persistently low levels of FSH and LH.
E Plasma cortisol levels are elevated.

210 With regard to the treatment of choriocarcinoma

A single agent chemotherapy is the most appropriate therapy.
B HCG measurement in the cerebrospinal fluid is an important initial investigation.
C hypothermia is appropriate.
D successful chemotherapy is followed by the return of fertility in most young women.
E actinomycin D is not an appropriate chemotherapeutic agent.

Illustrated case histories

Case 211

Mrs D, aged 24 years, a nonsmoker and married for 5 years, conceived shortly after stopping oral contraception. She attended for booking at 12 weeks' gestation. There was no relevant medical or surgical history, but there was a history of twins on the paternal side only. General examination was normal. The patient's weight was 78.8 kg, her height 1.70 m, and blood pressure 130/100 mmHg, with normal urine. All the routine pregnancy tests were carried out and subsequently reported normal. An ultrasound taken is shown in **211a**.

1. (a) What does the scan reveal and what would you tell the mother?
   (b) What are the fetal and maternal risks?

An alphafetoprotein (AFP) test carried out at 16 weeks' gestation was 107 units/ml (3.56 Multiples of the Mean (MoM)).

2. (a) What is the significance of this?
   (b) Should it be repeated?

At 26 weeks a second ultrasound (**211b**) was performed to assess fetal growth.

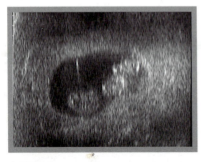

↑ **211a**

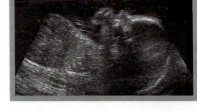

↑ **211b**

3. What does the scan show and what would you tell the mother?

The pregnancy continued uneventfully. At 38 weeks the head was engaged. Vaginal examination (VE) revealed the cervix to be partially effaced. It was decided to admit Mrs D for induction of labor.

4. Why do you think the consultant decided to induce labor?

At 0900 hrs an artificial rupture of the membranes (ARM) was carried out and clear liquor drained. A fetal scalp electrode was applied and a cardiotocograph (CTG) commenced. A syntocinon drip was started at 0915 hrs.

5. What instructions would you give to the midwives looking after this patient and when would you reassess her yourself?

At 1500 hrs you were requested to review the CTG (**211c**).

6. What does the CTG show?

At 1700 hrs the midwife carried out the VE to assess progress and found an abnormal presentation. You examine Mrs D and find the cervix is fully dilated and a face presentation left mentoanterior 1 cm below the ischial spines.

7. (a) What is your plan of action?
(b) How common is face presentation?
(c) What would you do if the position had been mentoposterior?

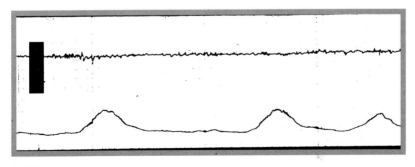

↑ **211c**

At 1715 hrs 'pushing' commenced but after 30 minutes Mrs D became distressed and the presenting part had not advanced. It was decided to carry out a forceps delivery using a pudendal block. A live male infant weighing 2950 g was delivered, with an Apgar score of 9 at 1 minute and 10 at 3 minutes. The placenta (**211d**) was delivered by controlled cord traction.

8. What does 211d reveal and what is the approximate incidence?

Puerperally Mrs D asked to breastfeed her baby.

9. Why is this often difficult with face presentation?

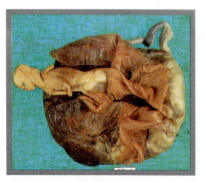

← **211d**

Case 212

Miss F, after visiting relations away from her home, presented as an emergency in labor. This was her first pregnancy and had, until then, been uneventful according to the maternity case records she carried with her. On examination she looked well and was not clinically anemic. Abdominal examination revealed a pregnant uterus compatible with her 36 weeks' gestation. There was a single fetus, longitudinal lie, with a breech presenting engaged in the pelvis; the fetal heart was regular. Clear fluid was noted to be coming from the vagina and, when tested with a nitrazine swab, it was confirmed to be liquor.

1. **What color would the nitrazine swab be if positive?**

On vaginal examination the cervix was 3 cm dilated and the findings were as shown in **212a**.

2. **(a)** **What type of breech presentation is it? How do you classify breech presentations?**
   (b) **What are the risks of this presentation?**

In view of the diagnosis, arrangements were made for an emergency Cesarean section under general anesthetic. Miss F was prepared for theater and on arrival in the anesthetic room was given sodium citrate, 30 ml, by mouth.

3. **(a)** **Why are antacids given to pregnant women in labor?**
   (b) **What other type of drugs are used?**

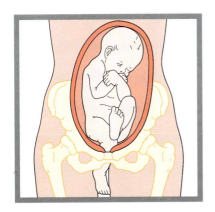

← **212a**

Anesthesia

Miss F was assisted on to the operating table and an intravenous infusion of Hartmann's solution commenced. Oxygen was given by face mask for 7 minutes, during which time the bladder was catheterized using aseptic technique. Anesthesia was induced with thiopental intravenously, followed by succinylcholine. Cricoid pressure was applied and the trachea intubated with a cuffed endotracheal tube.

4. (a) **What is the reason for applying cricoid pressure?**
(b) **Anesthesia is a cause of maternal death. What are some of the reasons for these deaths?**

A long-acting muscle relaxant was injected intravenously. The lungs were ventilated and anesthesia maintained with a mixture of nitrous oxide and halothane. During the operation intravenous papaveretum, 20 mg, was given for postoperative pain relief. Syntocinon, 10 units, was given intravenously following the delivery of the baby and, at the end of the operation, the muscle relaxant was reversed by using neostigmine and atropine.

Cesarean section

A transverse lower abdominal (Pfannenstiel) incision was made and the rectus sheath was incised transversely. The peritoneum of the uterovesical

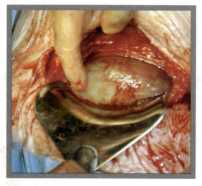

↑ **212b**

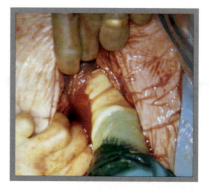

↑ **212c**

pouch was opened transversely above the bladder and separated from the uterus. A transverse incision was made in the lower segment until it was an adequate size to allow the delivery of the baby (**212b**).

5. (a) **What are the advantages of a transverse lower uterine segment incision over a vertical (classical) incision?**
   (b) **What are the chances of rupture of the respective uterine incisions in subsequent pregnancies?**
   (c) **When would you consider a 'classical' incision of the uterus to be justified?**

A hand was inserted into the uterine cavity (**212c**) below the breech (direct sacro-anterior); the right leg protruding through the cervical os was brought back into the uterine cavity and the breech delivered with the aid of external abdominal pressure from the assistant. Gentle groin traction was used to deliver the legs and the child as far as the umbilicus. Further traction allowed delivery of each arm in turn. A finger was placed in the baby's mouth to maintain flexion and, with pressure on the occiput, the head was delivered. The cord was clamped, then divided and the infant handed to the pediatrician (**212d**). The placenta was delivered by controlled cord traction after the intravenous oxytocin had been given (**212e**). The uterine cavity was explored to ensure that it was empty.

On opening the uterus an offensive smell had been noticed and a swab of the uterine cavity taken for culture and sensitivity.

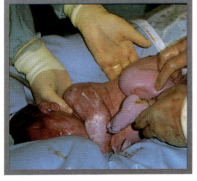

↑ **212d**

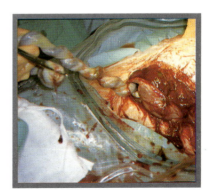

↑ **212e**

The uterus (**212f**) was closed in two layers and the uterovesical fold of peritoneum closed. Both fallopian tubes and ovaries were normal. The abdominal wall was closed in layers. The estimated blood loss was 750 ml.

6. (a) Should prophylactic pre- or intraoperative antibiotics be given routinely for all Cesarean section deliveries or only to selected cases?
   (b) If intraoperative antibiotics are given what would you recommend and why?

The baby

The female infant, weighing 2.75 kg, had Apgar scores of 2 at 1 minute, 5 at 3 minutes and 9 at 5 minutes. Resuscitation consisted of mucus extraction followed by intubation (**212g**) and intermittent positive pressure ventilation for 5 minutes. The endotracheal tube was removed and the baby cried spontaneously. The pediatrician considered that the baby should be kept under observation and therefore transferred to the special care baby unit (SCBU). On arrival in SCBU a full infection screen was performed. Vitamin K, 1 mg, was given intramuscularly. The following day, as the child was well, she was transferred to the ward to be with her mother.

Miss F was apyrexial on the first postoperative day, and had normal bowel sounds. On the second postoperative day she had a temperature of 38.4°C. Her lochia was noted to be offensive. A high vaginal swab (HVS) and

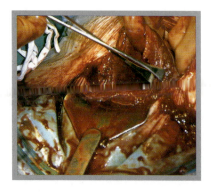

↑ **212f**

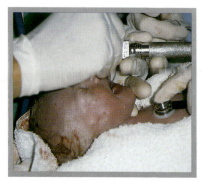

↑ **212g**

mid-stream specimen of urine (MSSU) was taken for culture. Beta-haemolytic streptococci were grown from both the intrauterine and the HVSs (taken during the operation) and the MSSU grew *Proteus mirabilis*. Intravenous ampicillin and metronidazole commenced. From then on Miss F made an uneventful recovery. Mother and baby 'bonded' well and they were discharged on the seventh day.

7. (a) What are the bacteria commonly responsible for infection after Cesarean section deliveries?
  (b) What are the two most common causes of failure to respond to antibiotic therapy?
  (c) What is the likely mode of delivery in the next pregnancy?

Case 213

Mrs M, aged 42 years, attended the outpatients department complaining that over the previous 4 months she had experienced 'spotting' and mid-cycle bleeding lasting for 2–3 days. Her periods were otherwise regular (3–4/28). She also noticed a 'lump coming down' the vagina, which caused a dragging sensation in the lower abdomen. There were no urinary or bowel symptoms.

Obstetric history: Five children, alive and well, aged between 20 and 8 years and their birth weights ranged from 2.8 to 4.0 kg. All vaginal deliveries, with her first child assisted by forceps.

Gynecological history: A cone biopsy because of CIN II/III 12 years previously. Completely excised and all subsequent smears normal.

On examination: Mrs M was well. The abdomen was soft and non-tender. On examination a large cystocele was noted (**213a**) and the cervix descended to the lower third of the vagina. The posterior vaginal wall was well supported. The uterus was normal size, mobile and retroverted. There were no adnexal masses.

1. (a) **What are the possible causes of intermenstrual bleeding in a woman aged 42?**
   (b) **Dilatation and curettage has been superseded by what procedure(s)?**

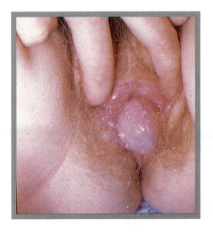

↑ **213a**

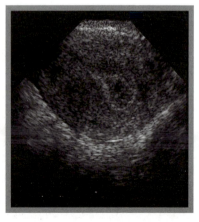

↑ **213b**

An endometrial polyp (**213b**) was found on ultrasound examination. Mrs M was admitted as a day case and the polyp removed at hysteroscopy (**213c**).

2. (a) What are the risks of hysteroscopy?
   (b) Are there any contraindications to hysteroscopy?

3. Is the endometrial polyp benign or malignant (213d)?

Follow-up at 6 weeks: There had been no further intermenstrual bleeding. Mrs J was well apart from the persistence of the dragging sensation in her lower abdomen, but did not wish any treatment at that time.
   Follow-up 4 months later: Mrs M's symptoms had increased in severity and she requested a repair operation and hysterectomy.

4. What specific questions should you ask a woman with a cystocele before a repair operation?

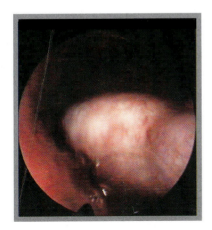

↑ **213c**

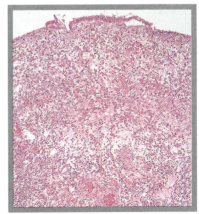

↑ **213d**

Operation under general anesthetic

Mrs M was placed in the lithotomy position. The anterior lip of the cervix was grasped with volsella, following which forceps were placed at 'Fothergill's points'.

5. (a) Who was Fothergill? Is it really necessary to identify these points?
(b) Some gynecologists use local infiltration (with or without epine-phrine) prior to carrying out a repair operation. Why?

The vaginal epithelium between these points and the urethra was incised and a triangular flap dissected from the underlying bladder. Blunt and sharp dissection was used to free the tissues behind the cervix. The pouch of Douglas was opened and the cardinal and uterosacral ligaments were identified. These were clamped and the pedicles doubly ligated on both sides. The uterine arteries were identified, clamped and ligated. The uterovesical peritoneum was defined and opened. The upper part of the broad ligament containing round ligament, ovarian ligament and fallopian tube was clamped and divided on both sides and the uterus removed. The ovaries appeared normal and were conserved. A purse-string suture closed the peritoneum, after which the left broad ligament pedicle was sutured to the right uterosacral ligament and vice versa (**213e**).

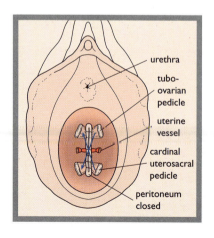

urethra

tubo-ovarian pedicle

uterine vessel

cardinal uterosacral pedicle

peritoneum closed

↑ **213e**

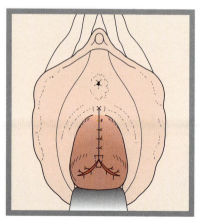

↑ **213f**

The pubocervical fascia was brought together in the midline, using interrupted sutures from below upwards, producing a support for the bladder neck and reducing the cystocele. The anterior vaginal wall was closed with interrupted sutures so that posteriorly the two angles allow for drainage and closure of the inverted V (**213f**). The vagina was packed and a Foley's catheter inserted into the bladder.

6. How long should the catheter remain *in situ*? What other alternatives are there for management of the bladder?

7. How common are enteroceles or vault prolapse after vaginal hysterectomy?

Postoperative course

In this case the pack was removed on the first day and the catheter removed on the third. A specimen of urine prior to its removal grew *Escherichia coli* and a course of co-trimoxazole tablets, 960 mg, twice daily for 7 days, was advised.
Mrs M was discharged on the fifth day.

8. Should preoperative or intraoperative antibiotics have been given if a catheter is left *in situ*?

Histology: The cervix showed mild chronic cervicitis. The endometrium was in the late secretory phase. Random sections from the myometrium showed no histological abnormality.
   Follow-up (8 weeks post-op): Mrs M was well. The 'dragging sensation' had disappeared. The anterior vaginal wall and vault had healed and there was no descent. She had no urinary symptoms and so was discharged.

Case 214

Mrs A, aged 30 years, height 1.67 m, weight 60 kg, complained of infertility of 3 years' duration. Her partner, aged 35, was 1.80 m in height and weighed 80 kg.

1. **What are the important features in the history of Mrs A and her partner that you need to obtain?**

2. **What examinations should be carried out, respectively, on Mrs A and her partner?**

You find nothing abnormal on examination of the couple and would have expected them to have conceived within 18 months.

3. **What features in the history or examination would make you consider that either Mrs A or her partner need special investigation as soon as possible?**

Investigations and results of tests carried out, or arranged, following first examination.			
Mrs A		**Partner**	
Day 21 progesterone:	29 nmol/l	Volume:	3 ml
Full blood count:	Normal	Concentration:	45 million/ml
Rubella status:	immune	Motility:	50%
Prolactin:	250 mU/l	Morphology:	50%
		semen analysis after 4 days' sexual abstinence	

4. The investigations in Table 1 were considered to be within normal limits. Do you agree?

A hysterosalpingogram (HSG) was carried out on Mrs A at the hospital.

5. One of these x-rays (214a-c) is Mrs A's HSG. Which one would you hope it is and why? What is your comment about the other two?

In view of the HSG finding, it was decided to carry out a laparoscopy, with hydrotubation with methylene blue. Mrs A's laparoscopy findings revealed normal pelvic organs and a free spill of dye.

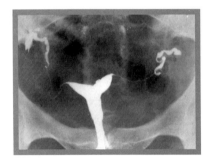

↑ **214a**

↑ **214b**

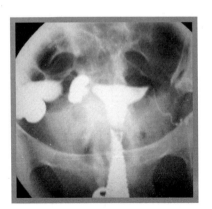

← **214c**

Mrs A had not conceived 1 year later so it was decided to stimulate ovulation. Figures **214d–i** reflect induction of ovulation and the variable response associated with clomiphene therapy and gonadotrophin administration on days 1, 3, and 5 of follicle stimulating hormone (FSH) and on day 8 of human chorionic gonadotrophin (HCG).

6. **Figure 214d shows a different response to 50 mg clomiphene citrate given on days 6–10 compared with successful conception on the third course of treatment (214e). How do you explain this?**

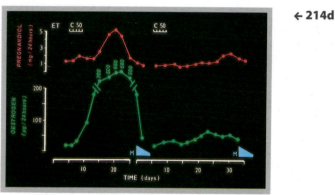

← **214d**

← **214e**

7. Figure **214f** shows the response to clomiphene and progesterone and Figure **214g** shows the response to gonadotrophins. What is the explanation for the respective responses?

Unfortunately Mrs A had no success with clomiphene (**214d**), so it was decided to use gonadotrophins in an era before downregulation techniques. After two courses of FSH on days 1, 3, and 5 and HCG on day 8, Mrs A conceived with results similar to **214g**. She had a normal pregnancy and delivery of a liveborn male infant, birth weight 3.2 kg.

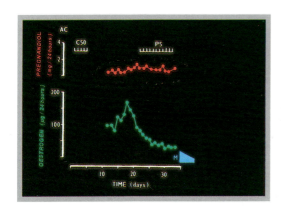

← **214f**

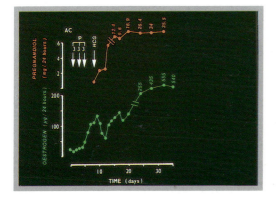

← **214g**

For comparison purposes only

A woman whose pituitary gland had been eradicated for a pituitary tumor in her teens had amenorrhea for 10 years prior to trying to achieve a pregnancy with gonadotrophins.

8. **What is your opinion of the two courses of FSH/HCG treatment in 214h and the two courses of FSH/HCG in 214i?**

← **214h**

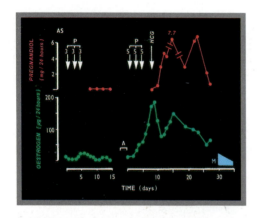

← **214i**

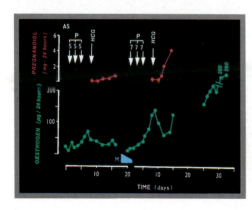

Case 215

Vulval soreness and pruritus vulvae are recognized gynecological symptoms but the etiology can be very different. The following three case histories are associated with a varied appearance of the vulva.

(A)
Mrs M, aged 64 years, had had pruritus vulvae for 5 years. The skin appeared red and 'eczematous' (**215a**) and she noticed that the skin 'weeps' at times. A routine cervical smear was difficult to interpret (possibly atrophic, possibly dyskaryotic) and, when repeated after topical estrogen, the smear confirmed an atrophic normal smear.

(B)
Mrs C, aged 44 years, had had pruritus vulvae for 15 years (**215b**) and also as a young child. The vulva was sore on touching and she had superficial dyspareunia. Her identical twin had a similar problem. On examination, the skin of the vulva was thin, pale and fragile. She had similar areas on the arms and wrists. A routine cervical smear was normal.

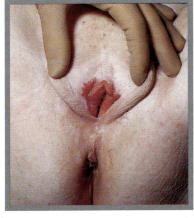

↑ **215a**

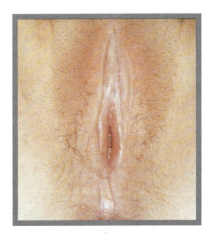

↑ **215b**

(C)
Miss F, aged 38 years, had had pruritus vulvae on and off for 5 years. The vulval appearance showed some thickened areas and some red, sore-looking areas (**215c**). She had previously had vulval warts in her teens. A routine cervical smear showed borderline nuclear changes.

1. What is the most likely clinical diagnosis for each of these cases (Mrs M, Mrs C and Ms F)?

2. Which of the following options do you think most reflects the appropriate management option for each of these women?
   (a) Excision biopsy of all abnormal skin.
   (b) Punch biopsy initially and, depending on report, removal of all abnormal skin.
   (c) Clinical diagnosis and single punch biopsy followed by treatment with bland emollients.

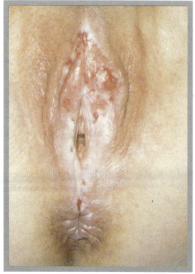

↑ **215c**

The so-called 'vulval dystrophies' are classified as follows: neoplastic and non-neoplastic
Neoplastic
Squamous Melanocytic Adenocarcinoma in situ
Non-neoplastic
Squamous epithelial hyperplasia lichen simplex lichen sclerosus other dermatoses

The histological appearances of lichen sclerosus (**215d**) and Paget's disease (**215e**) of the vulva are shown for comparison purposes.

3. What is the etiology of Paget's disease of the vulva?

4. If Mrs M developed a vulval 'lump' what diagnosis would you consider? Would you change your management?

5. If Mrs C was to develop areas of epithelial thickening, would this alter your management? If it would, what would you do? If it would not, justify the continuation of your previous management.

6. Is there any relationship between the borderline nuclear changes in Ms F's smear, the appearance of the vulva and the history of vulval warts in her teens?

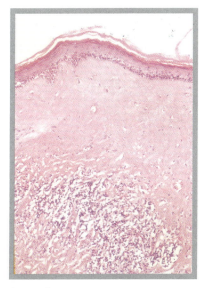

↑ **215d**

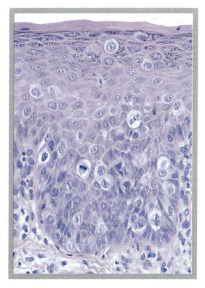

↑ **215e**

7. Following treatment Ms F presented with a lump adjacent to the anal margin. What would you do?

All three women developed carcinoma of the vulva or anus over a period of time, similar to the carcinoma depicted in **215f**.

8. How has the treatment of carcinoma of the vulva changed over the past 2–3 decades? What is the treatment for carcinoma of the anus?

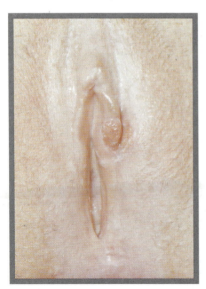

↑ **215f**

Case 216

Ms W, when aged 29 years, complained of heavy painful irregular periods. Her menstrual cycle was 7–14/21–28. She passed clots and used 10 pads per day during her periods. The pain was severe enough to stop her going to work.

She had not conceived during 4 years of unprotected intercourse. As a child she had an appendicectomy and 5 years previously she had had a laparoscopy because of unexplained lower abdominal and left iliac fossa pain. No cause was found but a pea-sized fibroid was seen at the fundus of the uterus. A diagnosis of spastic colon was made and her symptoms were relieved by ispaghula husk (Fybogel) and a high fibre diet.

After examination it was decided that Ms W should take a combined oral contraceptive pill for 3 months because of her menstrual symptoms. When reviewed 4 months later there was no real improvement in her symptoms. A laparoscopy was carried out and the findings are shown in **216a**.

1. The fibroid was partly subserous and 3–4 cm in diameter. Do you think it was a reason for her failure to conceive?

The fimbrial ends of both tubes, not shown in **216a**, appeared normal. There were a few filmy adhesions adjacent to the left ovary and a small area of 'active' endometriosis seen on the left uterosacral ligaments.

2. Could this be the reason why Ms W had not conceived?

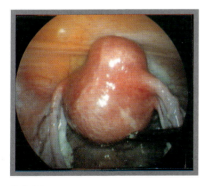

↑ **216a**

It was decided to prescribe danazol 200 mg t.d.s for 6 months. During this time, and for some months afterwards, Ms W's periods were reasonable and she led a normal life. Her previous stable relationship broke up and she married a man who had a child in his previous marriage. After 2 years of marriage Ms W had not conceived and she and her husband requested investigation of their infertility. Examination revealed that the fibroid had grown bigger and it was confirmed by ultrasound (**216b**) that there was more than one fibroid present. Clinically there was no evidence of endometriosis. The couple had the routine investigations carried out. The semen analysis was normal and ovulation was confirmed.

3. Is it justifiable to recommend a myomectomy operation?

No pregnancy occurred in the subsequent year so the couple requested that Ms W have an operation.

4. Would you give any treatment prior to the operation?

5. What is regarded as routine advice to women having a myomectomy operation? Is it appropriate?

When aged 33 years, Ms W had a laparotomy and a predominantly sub-serous fibroid 7 x 7 cm in diameter was removed from the fundus and back of the uterus, plus a small one on the anterior wall and a third subserous one in the right broad ligament.

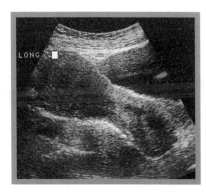

↑ **216b**

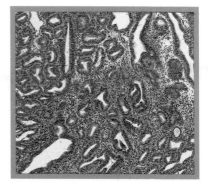

↑ **216c**

6. Should the uterine cavity be opened?

When aged 35 years, Ms W conceived and had a normal and uneventful pregnancy and normal vaginal delivery.

7. Approximately what proportion of women who have a myomectomy operation subsequently conceive?

Three years after the pregnancy Ms W's periods gradually deteriorated and interfered with her daily routine. An endometrial biopsy **(216c)** revealed endometrial hyperplasia, for which danazol was prescribed.

8. What type of endometrial hyperplasia is associated with the risk of neoplasia?

The features of endometrial hyperplasia following danazol therapy are shown in **216d**. It was decided, because of side effects of the danazol and failure to control the menstrual irregularities, to put her on medroxy-progsterone acetate, 200 mg/day. The change following 6 months of this progestogen therapy is revealed in **216e**. When aged 40 years, Ms W and her husband decided that, in view of the continued menstrual problems and histological findings, a hysterectomy was considered appropriate as their family was complete.

9. Would you conserve or remove the ovaries?

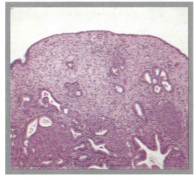

↑ **216d**

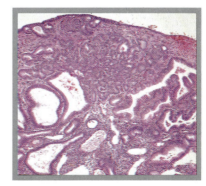

↑ **216e**

Case 217

Not all malignant or potentially malignant tumors have a poor prognosis, as illustrated by the two following cases who would be expected to survive.

Mrs S, aged 21 years, attended because she had been found to have an 'ovarian cyst' when attending for a routine cervical smear. An ultrasound scan was taken and is shown in **217a**.

1. (a) What is the mass likely to be?
(b) Are there any appropriate tumor markers?

Prior to reaching a decision as to what should be done about this cyst, Mrs S thought she might be pregnant. This was confirmed by a beta-human chorionic gonadotrophin (HCG) blood test. Mrs S and her husband were very anxious to have the baby and would not consider a termination of pregnancy because of their religious beliefs.

2. Was this a reasonable request? If yes, what advice would you give?

At 22 weeks, Mrs S had an episode of severe abdominal pain. As no specific diagnosis could be made it was considered that it was probably related to the ovarian tumor. At 23 weeks' gestation a laparotomy and left salpingo-oophorectomy was carried out as there was evidence of torsion of the ovarian cyst. The other ovary appeared to be normal. There was no free fluid present or any evidence of malignancy.

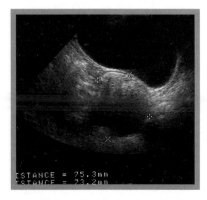

↑ **217a**

The pathologist confirmed that the ovarian tumor was an immature teratoma and contained neuroepithelial tissue (**217b**).

3. What additional information from the pathologist do you require and is torsion a recognized feature of these tumors?

Mrs S made a good recovery from her laparotomy and was discharged home on the sixth postoperative day. The remainder of her pregnancy was uneventful and she delivered her child, birth weight 3.25 kg, normally.

6 weeks: postnatal examination. No pelvic abnormality detected.

8 weeks: reviewed by a medical oncologist. In view of the histology report, Grade 2 with a fair amount of neuroepithelium, it was agreed to carry out an alphafetoprotein (AFP) estimation and arrange for a computerized axial tomography (CAT) scan. The CAT scan and AFP test were normal.

4. The prognosis for these tumors has improved in the last 3 decades and there are acknowledged effective chemotherapeutic regimes. Do you think:
   (i)   it is appropriate to adopt a policy of 'wait and see' with regular follow-up and AFP estimation; or
   (ii) is it preferable to give 6 courses of VAC (vincristine, doxorubicin, and cyclophosphamide) or another acceptable combination chemotherapy at 4-week intervals?

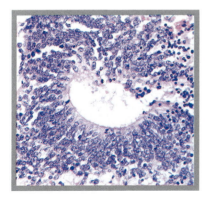

↑ **217b**

Three years after the pathological diagnosis, Mrs S is alive and well with no evidence of any recurrence. Any further pregnancies were to be delayed for 2 years.

Mrs U, when aged 52 years (4 years after her menopause), had vague abdominal symptoms and was found to have a large smooth swelling arising out of the pelvis (**217c**).

5. What is the gynecological differential diagnosis?

There was no evidence of any ascites. The mass appeared to be arising from the right ovary as the uterus was normal size and the left ovary was easily palpable. She had had no pregnancies deliberately and had been using oral contraception or condoms throughout her married life. A vaginal and Doppler ultrasound examination was carried out (**217d**).

6. What does the ultrasound show?

The preoperative CA 125 result was 69 IU/ml (normal level: 35 IU/ml). A laparotomy using a midline incision was carried out. There was no free fluid, so peritoneal washings were taken before removing the uterus and both ovaries. There was no evidence of abnormality in the omentum, appendix, peritoneal cavity, or on the diaphragm, and the liver was normal. An

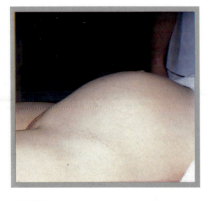

↑ **217c**

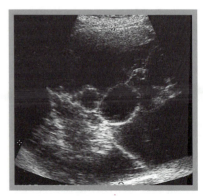

↑ **217d**

infracolic omentectomy was carried out and peritoneal washings were taken before closing the abdomen.

Pathology report

A borderline ovarian tumor. There was no evidence of any involvement of the cyst wall, but there was a solid nodule within the cystadenoma, which was borderline in nature.

The subsequent postoperative progress was uneventful and Mrs U was discharged on the seventh postoperative day.

7. (a)   What is your plan of action now?
   (b)   What is the recurrence rate for borderline mucinous (217e) and serous (217f) ovarian tumors?

When Mrs U attended for follow-up, she asked if she could go on hormone replacement therapy (HRT). The CA 125 level was 16 IU/ml and CT scan was normal. This scan would be used as the baseline for future comparisons.

8. What is your advice regarding HRT? Yes or no, and if yes what type?

It was agreed that the follow-up would be for at least 10 years by tumor markers (CA 125) and CT scan when considered appropriate.

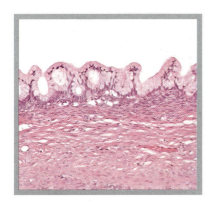

↑ **217e**

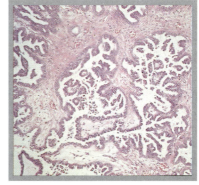

↑ **217f**

Case 218

The treatment of young women with invasive carcinoma of the cervix who have an intense desire for children is debatable. Four cases treated in the past 2 years illustrate some of the issues posed. The purpose of these brief case histories is to indicate some of the options, compared with a fifth woman who was aged 20 years when treated 12 years ago.

Ms A, aged 31 years and in a stable relationship, had a child by a previous partner. A smear taken 2 years previously was normal. She had complained of postcoital and intermenstrual bleeding for 2 months. Examination by her primary care practitioner revealed a large suspected carcinoma of the cervix. When seen, the lesion was a polypoidal tumour 3 x 3 cm in size, confined to the anterior lip of the cervix. An intraoperative picture of the tumor is shown in **218a**. There was no extension into the vaginal fornices and a rectal examination revealed no involvement of the parametrium or pelvic side walls.

1. (a) **What procedure could you carry out in the outpatients department?**
   (b) **Are there any investigations you would wish to arrange before deciding the most appropriate staging and treatment?**

Ms B, aged 30 years and also in a stable relationship, had had a cone biopsy, which revealed an adenocarcinoma of the cervix that was too large to classify as a microinvasive lesion.

2. **What are the limits of size and volume of carcinoma under the FIGO classification for Stage 1a and 1b?**

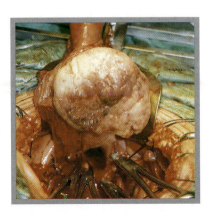

← 218a

Review of the pathology slides confirmed that the tumor must be staged as 1b and there was lymphatic involvement. Ms B requested another cone biopsy because of her and her partner's intense desire for a pregnancy.

3. Do you think that is justified?

The second cone biopsy revealed a single isolated small microscopic area of carcinoma. There was no evidence of lymphatic involvement and there was a wide resection margin.

4. What would you suggest as a plan of management if all options are available for detailed imaging techniques and in-vitro fertilization (IVF) treatment?

Ms C, aged 21 years and engaged, had a large (4 x 4 cm) Stage 1b carcinoma of the cervix. This was diagnosed after a 3-month history of postcoital bleeding. A computerized tomography (CT) scan indicated that there were enlarged nodes on the pelvic side walls. Ms C wanted to have a pregnancy of her own in the future and preferred surgery to radiotherapy and insisted on a Pfannenstiel incision. When the Wertheim's hysterectomy and lymphadenectomy were carried out, the large node at bifurcation of the right internal and external iliac blood vessels (shown partially freed in **218b**) was positive for tumor, as were two small paracervical nodes on the left side. All the other 30 lymph nodes removed were free of tumor.

5. What is the risk of carcinoma of the cervix occurring in the ovaries and where should the ovaries, if conserved, be placed?

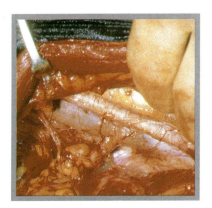

← **218b**

Ms D, aged 29 years, was referred for a Wertheim's hysterectomy after a cone biopsy had confirmed the presence of a multifocal Stage 1a carcinoma of the cervix incompletely excised. When seen, it was apparent that she was 10 weeks pregnant. She requested a second cone biopsy before she would consider radical surgery. A magnetic resonance imaging (MRI) scan was carried out and revealed no involvement of the pelvic wall lymph nodes.

6. What additional risks are there of a cone biopsy in pregnancy?

There were small areas of microinvasive carcinoma present in the second cone, but the resection margins were well free of tumor. It was decided by Ms D, after full discussion with her and her partner, that she would continue with the pregnancy. The top of the second cone biopsy was close to the internal os so at 14 weeks' gestation a cervical suture was inserted under anesthesia. At 26 weeks' gestation another MRI scan was carried out and no evidence of tumor seen. At 33–34 weeks. Ms D had a Cesarean section delivery and Wertheim's hysterectomy was carried out (**218c** and **218d**).

7. Is this appropriate treatment? Are there any additional risks in carrying out a radical hysterectomy after delivery of the child?

In 1980 Ms E, aged 17, Caucasian and a smoker, had a legal abortion at 10 weeks' gestation. A cervical smear at this time was normal. When aged 20 years she attended a Family Planning Clinic and a cervical smear was reported as normal. Seven months later she attended her primary care practitioner because of a bloodstained discharge. The smear taken was

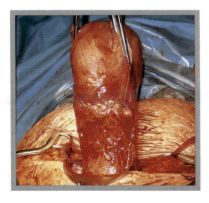

↑ **218c**

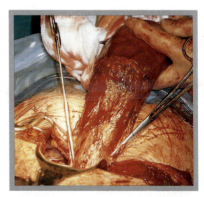

↑ **218d**

'abnormal, refer for colposcopy'. Colposcopy revealed a small area of aceto-white on Schiller positive areas at the 5 o'clock position of the cervix. Smears from the ecto- and endocervical canal were suspicious of a clear cell adenocarcinoma. Biopsies from the abnormal area of the cervix revealed a multifocal clear cell carcinoma. There was no history of her mother taking estrogens in pregnancy. The CT scan findings are shown in **218e** and **218f**.

Initially an extraperitoneal approach was used to remove lymph nodes from the external and internal iliac and along both common iliac blood vessels. They and the obturator nodes were sent for frozen section. All were reported as negative. A Wertheim's hysterectomy and pelvic lympha-denopathy were carried out. The fallopian tubes were removed and both ovaries conserved.

8. What is the reasoning behind removing the fallopian tubes?

Ms E made a good recovery following her radical hysterectomy and was counselled regarding the need to be followed up regularly. After the first 5 years of regular follow-up Ms E, who was now married, enquired about the possibility of IVF and a surrogate pregnancy. This was arranged and at the third attempt a successful IVF surrogate multiple pregnancy using her ova and her husband's sperm was achieved. She is now alive and well (as are her children)12 years after her radical hysterectomy.

9. (a) Was Ms E over treated?
    (b) What are the chances of the 4 other young women surviving 12 years?

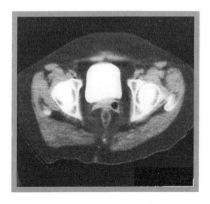

↑ 218e

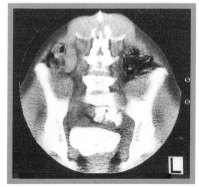

↑ 218f

Case 219

Mrs P was booked for hospital delivery in her first pregnancy, which was uneventful. She had a normal delivery of a male infant. An episiotomy was repaired by the midwife. It apparently broke down after discharge from hospital and she was given antibiotics. Mrs P returned for her 6-week postnatal check. She complained of having frequent and recurrent vaginal discharges. On examination there was vaginal discharge present and a swab taken for culture.

1. What is the most likely cause of the vaginal discharge?

It was obvious on inspection that there was a gross deficiency of the perineum and that the vaginal introitus was extremely close to the anus depicted diagramatically in **219a**.

Further questioning revealed that the episiotomy scar had become infected 2 days after discharge from hospital. The 'episiotomy' healed after a month. In the meantime her persistent vaginal discharge was treated with clotrimazole pessaries and cream and further antibiotics. Mrs P had noted that her anus was very close to the vagina because she had symptoms of fecal urgency and now opened her bowels four to five times a day.

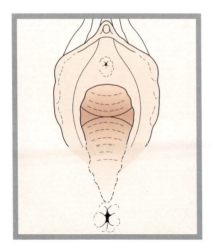

↑ **219a**

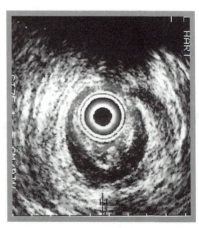

↑ **219b**

2. What other examination would be essential in this postnatal visit?

A detailed study of anorectal function was carried out (**219b**).
When her child was 7 months old, Mrs P was brought in for repair of the
perineum and her levator ani.

3. What preoperative preparations should be made?

At operation, careful dissection exposed the torn levator ani and the
sphincter ani. The sphincter ani muscles were sutured together with
interrupted vicryl sutures, and the levator ani supported with separate
sutures, depicted diagramatically in **219c**.
   At the end of the operation, vaginal and rectal examinations showed
considerable improvement of the sphincter ani. Intraoperative antibiotics
were given. When reviewed 3 months later Mrs P's bowel symptoms were
much improved, but further detailed anorectal studies indicated that the
sphincter still needed further tightening. The anal sphincter was still
deficient anteriorly and there was too narrow a gap in the perineum
between the vaginal orifice and the anus. It was decided to review the
situation in 3–4 months.

4. Was this a reasonable decision?

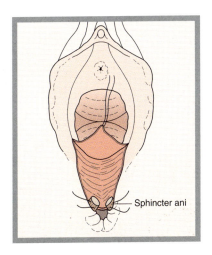

Sphincter ani

↑ **219c**

When admitted 8 months after her previous operation, Mrs P had no tenderness, diarrhea, constipation, dyspareunia, dysmenorrhea, intermenstrual bleeding, or postcoital bleeding. She did, however, state that she felt her 'vaginal muscles' during coitus were still weaker than before her pregnancy.

At operation, skin was incised posterior to the vaginal introitus; the levator muscles were again exposed, and built up and approximated. A skin flap was excised from the left side of the vulva and placed over the area between the vaginal orifice and the anus (**219d**). The perineum was there-fore bridged by the skin flap. The two margins of the flap were sutured and the vulval margins sutured together (**219e**) and the donor site was also sutured.

5. What other type of skin graft might have been used to build up the perineum?

One year later Mrs P became pregnant. Because of her previous unpleasant experience she wished to be delivered by Cesarean section and this was agreed. At Cesarean section she was delivered of a female infant weighing 2980 g and she was discharged home on the fifth day.

6. What other types of perineal or vaginal operations would justify delivery by Cesarean section?

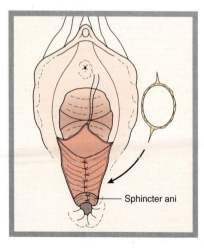

— Sphincter ani

↑ **219d**

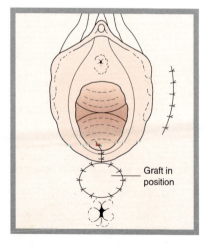

Graft in position

↑ **219e**

Picture Tests Answers

1   **(a)** It was taken because the mother had symptoms suggestive of urinary calculi and under these circumstances it is important to establish the diagnosis. This should be done as quickly as possible, with the minimum risk to the fetus, by a single plain radiograph and a single 20-minute intravenous urogram (IVU) film if ultrasound fails to make the diagnosis. Unnecessary delay may result in irreversible damage to the maternal kidney owing to septic obstruction or result in premature labor secondary to renal colic and/or sepsis.
(b) Most women complain of pain in the loin or flank, and many have urinary tract infection and sepsis arising from obstruction of the urinary tract. This can result in septicemia.
(c) The renal calculus is passed spontaneously with conservative management comprising bed rest, hydration, analgesia, and antibiotics as indicated. Fortunately, the majority of cases occur in the second or third trimester of pregnancy and, therefore, the risks to the fetus of radiation are less than in the first trimester.
(d) Open invasive techniques have been replaced in most cases by cystoscopic stent replacement, percutaneous insertion of a stent, or ureteroscopy and stone extraction. The use of lithotripsy, which is well established in the nongravid woman, is contraindicated in pregnancy.

2   **(a)** This was a secondary melanoma tumor. It could, however, represent a secondary tumor from the cervix, endometrium, or kidney.
(b) Excision biopsy.
(c) This is a difficult problem because melanoma has a very poor prognosis. Imaging techniques, such as magnetic resonance imaging (MRI) or computerized tomography (CT) scans, could be used to see whether there was disease elsewhere. Since the prognosis is poor and chemotherapy does not offer a great deal of help, one hopes that local excision is curative. In this case the patient had melanoma in the pelvis and further surgery and palliateive chemotherapy were required.
(d) The liver.

3   **(a)** No, there may well be a double genital tract and there may be an associated renal abnormality.
(b) Problems with the delivery; particularly, it may be traumatized or may have to be divided in order to achieve a satisfactory vaginal delivery.
(c) If there is an associated double genital tract some of these women may complain of dysmenorrhea. Complete septums of the vagina can be easily missed, particularly using a bivalve speculum, since the septum can be pushed to one side and not recognized.
(d) There is potential risk of damage to the bladder and to the rectum.

4   **(a)** Carcinoma of the vagina.
(b) A posterior exenteration.
(c) If the pelvic lymph nodes are all negative then the chances of success for this type of procedure would be in the order of 35–50%.
(d) There should be no evidence of disease outside the pelvis on imaging techniques. The patient should be reasonably fit for her age. She should be able to cope with a permanent

105

colostomy and absence of vagina or the formation of a neovagina from bowel and be able to withstand the physical and psychological effects of this major surgery. There is also the question of her partner adapting to the changed circumstances.

5 **(a)** The most likely diagnosis is female pseudohermaphroditism. These individuals usually present with ambiguous genitalia at birth but the disorder may not be detected for several years.
(b) The three most common adrenal enzyme defects are 21-hydroxylase deficiency, 11-beta-hydroxylase deficiency and 3-beta-hydroxysteroid dehydroxylase deficiency. All these result in increased androgen production in utero and consequent virilization of the external genitalia. These enzyme defects result in a reduced cortisol secretion, with increased pituitary adrenocorticotrophic hormone (ACTH) and, in consequence, adrenal androgen overproduction.
(c) All types of congenital adrenal hyperplasia are transmitted as an autosomal trait.
(d) Replacement therapy with exogenous corticosteroid therapy is indicated in all affected forms of congenital adrenal hyperplasia (CAH). Mineralocorticoid as well as glucocorticoid replacement is needed in some forms of CAH. In addition, surgery may be necessary to produce reasonable appearances of the external genitalia. All these individuals are 46XX individuals and ovaries are present.

6 **(a)** Placenta accreta occurs when there is pathological adherence due to the paucity of underlying decidua. Placenta increta is, where the placenta invades the uterine wall, and placenta percreta is, where the invasion reaches the uterine serosa and may even lead to rupture of the uterus.
(b) In over 50% of cases it is associated with placenta previa, possibly because of a deficiency of the decidua in the lower uterine segment. Any condition resulting in a reduction of decidua can lead to either partial or complete abnormal adherence, so it can include multiparity, previous infection, uterine scar, or previous traumatic curettage.
(c) The lowest mortality has been reported to be associated with an immediate hysterectomy. The conservative approach of tying off the placental cord and leaving the placenta in situ in the uterus (if there has been no excessive bleeding) and awaiting its slow absorption is no longer felt to be appropriate, unless it is considered necessary for a young patient to retain her fertility at all costs.
(d) They are related to infection and hemorrhage that may occur at any time. Lactation does not occur and the woman remains amenorrheic for 12–18 months.

7 **(a)** Either a fibroid or a solid ovarian tumor, such as a dysgerminoma.
(b) In the case of a fibroid, it certainly should be curative. If it is an ovarian dysgerminoma, for example, then the results may also be good as it is very sensitive to subsequent radiotherapy or chemotherapy. The advantage of chemotherapy, of course, is that it may allow fertility to be retained if the tumor is unilateral and there is no evidence of any recurrence after treatment. If the tumor is ovarian, it does depend on whether the lesion is confined to one ovary or present in both ovaries. In the latter case, radical treatment will be appropriate. If it was a nongerm cell tumor then it would be treated in a similar manner to epithelial ovarian cancers.
(c) Germ cell tumor.
(d) If it was a fibroid, then it is possible as recurrence is not uncommon.

8 **(a)** Yes, by ultrasound.

(b) Termination of pregnancy.

(c) A Cesarean section delivery is the usual mode of delivery and preterm Cesarean section is usually recommended. The use of steroids to stimulate surfactant production is advisable and nowadays many obstetricians would favour elective delivery at 37 weeks or earlier.

(d) Some obstetricians recommend a classical incision, but this would seem to offer little fetal benefit over the lower segment incision or a vertical incision starting in the lower segment, but it does increase the maternal risks, particularly of uterine scar rupture in any subsequent pregnancy.

9   **(a)** Trichomonas infection of the cervix.

(b) Metronidazole 200 mg t.d.s. for 7–10 days.

(c) Premenopausal. The clear cervical mucus also suggests that it is from a patient midcycle.

(d) Because there is constant reinfection from an infected partner. Both the woman and her partner(s) should be treated at the same time and sometimes barrier contraception is recommended temporarily to avoid reinfection.

10   **(a)** An X-ray with a Lippes loop.

(b) Outside.

(c) If practical by laparoscopy, but it may require to removal by laparotomy.

(d) The incidence is uncommon but not rare. Perforation of the uterine corpus or fundus has been reported to range from 1 to 350 to 2,500. The incidence of cervical perforation has been suggested to be about 3–10 per 1,000 insertions.

11   **(a)** Genital herpes.

(b) About 90%.

(c) A watery vaginal discharge, which may be profuse. The presence of intranuclear inclusion bodies and multinucleated vaginal cells in a cervical smear implies infection with herpes simplex virus.

(d) There are currently no agents that completely eradicate the herpes simplex virus. However, the antiviral agent acyclovir, administered orally and intravenously, shortens the duration of symptoms and the viral shedding and/or decreases the incidence of new lesion formation and extragenital symptoms in patients with primary infections.

12   **(a)** A full bladder, in this patient in the second stage of labor.

(b) It might be associated with a malpresentation or cephalopelvic disproportion.

(c) Simply to catheterize the woman and possibly leave an indwelling catheter in situ, depending on the presentation.

(d) No.

13   **(a)** Filshie clips.

(b) Menstrual problems.

(c) Yes, from the appearance of the tubes. Although one cannot see the fimbriated end of each tube it would seem to be suitable for a reversal operation by removal of the clips and tubo-tubal reanastomosis.

(d) The clips are inert, but many gynecologists do remove the part of the tube containing the clip as long as it does not interfere with the blood supply of the ovaries.

14   **(a)** The diagnosis is a procidentia with carcinoma of the vagina. One could do a vaginal hysterectomy excising the large lesion and possibly consider radiotherapy afterwards, depending on the histopathological findings.

(b) Possibly chronic irritation. It may be associated with prolonged (or neglected) use of a ring pessary. Nowadays it would be expected to be diagnosed at an earlier stage if pessaries are replaced at regular intervals.

(c) An intravenous pyelogram and either a CT or a magnetic resonance imaging (MRI) scan.

(d) If technically easy. A Schauta type of operation with removal of the ovaries is appropriate. A vaginal hysterectomy and external radiotherapy is another possibility.

15 **(a)** There is marked vascularity and considerable hirsutism.

(b) This is quite often characteristic of Stein–Leventhal (polycystic ovary) syndrome, where there is increased vascularity of the breast and, in conjunction with their bouts of amenorrhea, it can mimic the changes seen in pregnancy.

(c) No, not unless the patient is anxious for pregnancy and treatment of her infertility.

(d) If she is above average weight then one might advise her to lose weight. Small doses of prednisolone may change the hormone imbalance or cyproterone and oestrogen (Dianette) may be given to regularize her periods. The long-term risks are of endometrial hyperplasia and, possibly, the development of endometrial carcinoma.

16 **(a)** Marked blood vessels beneath the skin, suggesting a collateral circulation.

(b) It might be secondary to deep venous thrombosis or, alternatively, it might be due to a collateral circulation as a consequence of hepatic cirrhosis, but in that condition the veins usually run vertically rather than transversely.

(c) This patient might well be on long-term oral anticoagulant therapy.

(d) Whether it is minor or major surgery it would be preferable for this patient to be anticoagulated with heparin.

17 **(a)** There appears to be an abnormal reddened area, which may well reflect VAIN III.

(b) Take smears and possibly vaginal biopsy.

(c) Aceto-white and Schiller negative areas plus abnormal vascular pattern.

(d) She may develop a vaginal carcinoma so she needs regular follow-up.

18 **(a)** It shows a small cyst just below the urethra and it could represent a Gartner's duct remnant.

(b) Benign.

(c) By marsupializing or excising this.

(d) With appropriate treatment it should not recur. Marsupialisation would allow the basal epithelium to be epithelialized with vaginal epithelium and it would not be noticeable in a few weeks. Excision may be associated with considerable bleeding and hematoma formation. It is not likely to recur by either operative technique.

19 **(a)** This is a placenta with hydatidiform mole. The treatment is that this patient be followed up by human chorionic gonadotrophin (HCG) estimations and should avoid a pregnancy for 1–2 years.

(b) Complete mole currently occurs in approximately 1 in 1500 pregnancies in the UK and USA.

(c) 46XX, although the vast majority of partial hydatidiform moles have a triploid karyotype, usually 69XXY, but occasionally it is 69XXX or 69XYY.

(d) It is a very rare complication. It occurs in about 1 in 50,000 gestations, 50% of which follow a molar pregnancy, 30% follow an abortion or ectopic gestation, and 20% follow an apparently normal pregnancy.

20 **(a)** Yes, the common abnormalities of Turner's syndrome include epicanthal folds, high arched palate, low nuchal hairline, webbed neck, shield-like chest, coarctation of the aorta, ventricular septal defect, renal abnormalities, pigmented nevi, lymphedema, hyperplastic nails, cubitus valgus, inverted nipples, and double eyelashes may be present as well. However, no feature individually is absolutely pathognomonic.
(b) Usually 45XO, but a number of different abnormalities of the X chromosome are associated with gonadal dysgenesis.
(c) Primary amenorrhea, but short stature is another common reason for which advice is sought.
(d) FSH and LH levels would be increased and there would be streak gonads.

21 **(a)** A small inclusion cyst in the perineum.
(b) Excise it and send it for biopsy.
(c) No.
(d) Either congenital or foreign body/materials included in a time of previous surgery.

22 **(a)** Yes. Although it is perianal it is still considered in the vulval area.
(b) Excision biopsy.
(c) If the excision is not wide enough and the margins are not surgically clear then a further wider excision might be necessary. Assessment of the anus and lower rectum should be checked to make sure that there is no intraepithelial neoplasia there.
(d) It could be radiotherapy or a combination of radiotherapy and surgery. Surgery near the sphincter is a potential problem and radiotherapy, under the circumstances, may be preferable.

23 **(a)** Carcinoma of the cervix.
(b) Yes.
(c) Pelvic wall lymphadenectomy.
(d) Yes, if the nodes were involved then further treatment in the form of radiotherapy would be appropriate. There should be an 85–95% cure rate if the lymph nodes are not involved, but it may drop to 65–75% with the lymph nodes involved, assuming that postoperative radiotherapy is given.

24 **(a)** It reveals a urethral fistula.
(b) It may be a traumatic injury or a surgical injury.
(c) Since only half the length of the urethra is necessary, this X-ray suggests that it would be reasonable to remove the lower half of the urethra.
(d) No, it is a rare condition.

25 **(a)** Bilateral epithelial tumors.
(b) As the tumors seem to be multiloculated, it would probably be appropriate to carry out a total hysterectomy, bilateral salpingo-oophorectomy, and omentectomy, and, take washings of the peritoneal fluid before and after their removal.
(c) If malignant, the cure rate is probably only about 25–30% at the outside, despite chemotherapy. If borderline, then approximately 6% will recur and become malignant.
(d) Combination chemotherapy including cisplatin or carboplatin. There are developments with taxol, but it is expensive and in limited supply at the present time.

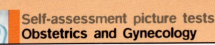

26 **(a)** Suction termination of pregnancy.
(b) (i) Continuing the pregnancy would involve risk to the life of the pregnant women greater than if the pregnancy was terminated.
(ii) The termination is necessary to prevent grave permanent injury to physical or mental health of the pregnant woman.
(iii) The pregnancy has not exceeded its 24th week and continuing with the pregnancy would involve risk, greater than if the pregnancy were terminated, of injury to the physical or mental health of the pregnant woman.
(iv) The pregnancy has not exceeded its 24th week and continuing with the pregnancy would involve risk, greater than if the pregnancy were terminated, of injury to the physical or mental health of any existing child(ren) of the family of the pregnant woman.
(v) There is a substantial risk that if the child was born it would suffer from physical or mental abnormalities as to be seriously handicapped.
(c) Yes, there is a risk of sepsis, infection, perforation, and incomplete removal of the products. Administration of prostaglandins to soften and dilate the cervix is appropriate.
(d) It is satisfactory without any complications.

27 **(a)** Melanoma of the abdominal wall and vulval area.
(b) Wide excision of the lesions.
(c) No, other than telling the patient that the lesion is completely excised and that she should contact you if there appears to be any occurrence of any pigmented areas, no particular follow-up is necessary.
(d) Probably not; because of the obvious obesity of the patient the skin should be easily freed and primary closure obtained.

28 **(a)** Second-degree uterine prolapse, but with traction on the cervix it may be a third-degree prolapse.
(b) Treatment would be a vaginal hysterectomy and anterior and posterior repair. The general health of the patient may be very poor and the prolapse may need to be controlled with a pessary. The operation could be done under local anesthesia, epidural, or spinal analgesia without particular problems so most patients can be operated on.
(c) The development of an enterocele, but with proper support this should not be common.
(d) In general, patients should be advised to take things easy and made to realize that they have had a hernia operation and that they need to take things easy (avoid heavy lifting and manual work) to allow for proper healing over a period of 2–3 months.

29 **(a)** Check FSH and LH levels and screen for androgen levels and possibly, if indicated, an ultrasound scan of the ovaries.
(b) Probably. It would probably be worthwhile giving the patient cyproterone acetate first of all or a pill with a higher estrogen level to see whether this improved her situation.
(c) Oral tetracycline and local application of retinoic acid preparations.
(d) Yes, if they are regular ovulatory menstrual cycles.

30 **(a)** It could be accounted for by failure of one Müllerian duct to develop.
(b) There is no contraindication to conception.
(c) Yes, in fact this patient did have only one kidney (on the same side) but there was no development at all on the opposite side of the Müllerian duct or kidney.
(d) It contained a pregnancy.

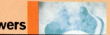

31 **(a)** Leukoplakia or vulval dystrophy are still used as the gynecological diagnosis, but dermatologists would regard it as lichen sclerosus.
(b) It looks as though there is a small ulcerated area and it may well be due to cracking or, possibly, a small early carcinoma may be present. There is also a midline lower abdominal scar.
(c) Malignancy should be excluded first by biopsy of the ulcerated areas. If positive or VIN III, then it could be treated surgically, but some skin grafting may be required. If negative, medical treatment would consist of bland ointments and occasional steroid cream if there is marked irritation.
(d) Diabetes mellitus is the most likely condition associated with vulval dystrophies. Other causes include anemia, deficiency states, and sensitivity or allergies.

32 **(a)** There is a tumor just below the urethra on the right side and possibly a smaller one on the left. There also is an abnormal area on the lower left side of the vagina by the speculum.
(b) This was a recurrent tumor following a hysterectomy for carcinoma of the endometrium.
(c) Obviously these tumor nodules need to be removed. It may be appropriate to excise them followed by radiotherapy. Alternatively, exenteration may be considered if there is no spread elsewhere. As endometrial carcinoma initially medroxyprogesterone acetate might be beneficial.
(d) The long-term prognosis is probably poor unless the tumors respond to excision, chemotherapy, or radiotherapy.

33 **(a)** It looks like a suburethral cyst or urethrocele and cystocele.
(b) If an urethral cyst, by excision and removal. If urethrocele and cystocele, by a repair.
(c) It is very likely to be benign.
(d) There are potential dangers to the urethra. There might even be a diverticulum, but one should be prepared to reconstitute the urethra if necessary.

34 **(a)** One cause is pre-eclampsia and another could be lymphedema following surgery.
(b) One would check the urine and blood pressure, as the patient may have pre-eclampsia.
(c) By firm bandaging for a few days and then application of special support stockings.
(d) Surgery of the vulva and interference with the lymphatic chain in the superficial and deep femoral and inguinal lymph glands.

35 **(a)** This is a velamentous placenta.
(b) Vasa praevia.
(c) Yes.
(d) Not commonly with retained placenta, but postpartum hemorrhage is likely if the vessels become detached in delivering the placenta.

36 **(a)** This is an ovarian ectopic pregnancy. A primary ovarian pregnancy is one in which the ovum is fertilized while still in the follicle or, if an ovum is fertilized outside the fallopian tube, implants primarily in the ovary. In secondary ovarian pregnancy the ovum is fertilized inside the tube and the conception extruded from the tube to implant on the ovary.
(b) Women using an intrauterine contraceptive device (IUCD), as these reduce tubal and uterine implantation.
(c) The fallopian tube must be normal and separate from the ovary, ovarian tissue must be identified histologically in the wall of the gestational sac, and the gestational sac must occupy the normal site of the ovary and be attached to the uterus by the ovarian ligament.
(d) Patients usually abort in the first trimester of pregnancy, but a few continue to term.

37 **(a)** She has had an episiotomy or tear on the right side. The healed scar is apparent. If an episiotomy, it was lateral rather than being mediolateral. There has obviously been marked healing, with granulation tissue at the introital area. There is also obvious loss of symmetry.
(b) A Fenton's operation.
(c) A 'Z' plasty.
(d) 95–100%.

38 **(a)** Vulval and perianal warts (condylomata acuminata).
(b) They are caused by the human papilloma virus (HPV) and can be sexually transmitted.
(c) Where there is immune impairment and spontaneous or iatrogenic diabetes mellitus. Women with poor perineal hygiene.
(d) They may grow very rapidly and extend into the whole of the vagina. It may be necessary to deliver the baby by Cesarean section.

39 **(a)** Vaginal ovoids and an intrauterine tube
(b) Previously radium, but for the past three decades cesium.
(c) Treating carcinoma of the cervix.
(d) Most likely Stage IB, II or III carcinoma of the cervix, but it could also be carcinoma of the body of the uterus. In the latter, there would be a larger dose in the intrauterine tube.

40 **(a)** Congenital hypertrophic pyloric stenosis.
(b) During the second or third month of life.
(c) Persistent, forceful ('projectile') vomiting after every meal.
(d) In mild cases, treatment with antispasmodics may be successful, but it is usual to operate and split the hypertrophied pyloric musculature longitudinally down to the mucosa (Ramstedt's operation).

41 **(a)** Fibroma.
(b) Most commonly 40–60 years of age.
(c) The vast majority are benign.
(d) Fluid may accumulate in the pleural cavity (in association with ascites leading to Meig's syndrome) and occasionally the anterior abdominal wall, vulva, or legs.

42 **(a)** Pain as the 'mass' is extruded through the cervix.
(b) Premenopausal as the ovaries are conserved.
(c) Submucous fibroid.
(d) Ureters near the cervix. Insert ureteric catheters prior to the hysterectomy, but even so they may be difficult to feel in the paracervical area.

43 **(a)** Cataract, therefore the diagnosis is toxoplasmosis.
(b) Maternal: IgG seroconversion, T-IgM.
Fetal/neonatal: Cord IgM, placental histology, abnormal cerebrospinal fluid (CSF).
(c) Chorioretinitis, fever, hydrocephaly, hepatosplenomegaly, thrombocytopenia, seizures. Long-term sequelae are mental retardation, severe visual defects, and seizures.
(d) Maternal screening is mandatory in France and Australia but, because of the low prevalence in the UK and USA, the high cost, and lack of reliability of serological testing, it is not considered appropriate at the present time.

44 **(a)** Pelvic tuberculosis, which is secondary to a focus of infection elsewhere.

(b) Pulmonary tuberculosis is the most common medical condition, or tuberculosis of other organs, e.g. the urinary tract.

(c) Infertility (with or without oligomenorrhea or amenorrhea) or ectopic pregnancy.

(d) Adenocarcinoma of the fallopian tube can be coexistent with tuberculosis, but endometrial atypia may be mistaken for carcinoma.

45 **(a)** Pregnancy-induced hypertension and diabetes mellitus.

(b) Diabetes mellitus.

(c) The fetal prognosis is adversely influenced because of higher perinatal wastage.

(d) The kidneys.

46 **(a)** Cryosurgery.

(b) Cervical ectopy and cervical intraepithelial neoplasia (CIN).

(c) Ectopies are often present (particularly if the patient is taking oral contraception) and the excess vaginal discharge is improved for a time. It can be appropriate treatment for mild degrees of CIN, but all cases need careful follow-up. Most failures are noted within 1 year. The overall failure rate is about 8%, irrespective of the grade of CIN. Its advantage is that it is an effective outpatient therapy and can be repeated and is virtually pain free.

(d) Patients are likely to have a watery discharge for 10–14 days and should avoid intercourse while the watery discharge is present.

47 **(a)** Following pelvic surgery, management of acute retention of urine, urethral trauma or surgery, or when there is acute vulvovaginal irritation and a urethral catheter would cause more discomfort.

(b) Advantages: the reduction of incidence of infection compared with urethral catheter, more comfortable for the patient, and easier for nursing staff to manage.

Disadvantages: it requires medical staff to insert and there is a risk of damage to other organs at the time of insertion.

(c) Contraindications include the inability to distend the bladder or if a recent cystostomy has been performed. Gross hematoma is also a contraindication if there is only a small-gauge catheter available.

(d) An immediate complication can be perforation of the large or small bowel. The equipment can block or may fracture and a portion of catheter may be retained in the bladder.

48 **(a)** It is related to the management of Rhesus (Rh) hemolytic disease and was introduced by Liley. It reflects one of the major developments in the management of a condition that was an important cause of stillbirth and fetal mortality and morbidity.

(b) Early in the 1960s.

(c) The development of anti-D immunoglobulin prophylaxis programmes

(d) Determine the Rhesus status of the woman. If Rh-negative, check the history regarding blood transfusions. Check for presence of antibodies in maternal serum. If antibodies are present check the partner's ABO blood group and Rhesus status and if he is Rh-positive determine his genotype and zygosity.

49 **(a)** Exomphalos (omphalocele).

(b) Maternal serum alphafetoprotein (AFP) screening and ultrasound screening.

(c) The most common variety is due to failure of the physiological hernia to return at 9 weeks' gestation.

(d) The prognosis depends on its size and contents. Although all may be amenable to surgery,

the association of malformations and/or postoperative complications may influence the
outcome

50 **(a)** *Neisseria gonorrhoeae*, small kidney-shaped Gram-negative cocci arranged in pairs.
(b) Endocervix, urethra, anorectum, and pharynx.
(c) Chlamydial infection.
(d) Penicillinase-producing strains of *N. gonorrhoeae*.

51 **(a)** No right kidney or ureter visible. Slight dilatation or hypertrophy of the left kidney and
lower ureter.
(b) It is uncommon, but a recognized congenital abnormality.
(c) Uterine abnormality. In fact this woman had a double uterus (see 61).
(d) There is a risk of urinary tract infection, and prophylactic antibiotic therapy may be
considered necessary for any delivery or operation.

52 **(a)** *Trichomonas vaginitis*.
(b) A flagellated protozoan organism.
(c) Microscopic examination of discharge or culture.
(d) Metronidazole 200 mg t.d.s. for 7–10 days and also treat the partner.

53 **(a)** It was associated with the toxic shock syndrome.
(b) It is uncertain whether they have an anti-implantation effect or there is an influence on
tubal function. If impregnated with progestogen, there is an additional hormonal effect.
(c) *Actinomyces*.
(d) The failure rate is 0.5–1% in any menstrual cycle or three to four pregnancies per 100
woman-years.

54 **(a)** A hip prosthesis. Various types have been produced since the original Charnley's design.
(b) Post menopausal, 65–75+ years.
(c) No, just a simple injury that resulted in a fractured neck of femur.
(d) Yes, by the administration of hormone replacement therapy just prior to or at the
menopause. Activity is also a factor.

55 **(a)** Pelvic infection, pain, dyspareunia, or menstrual problems.
(b) Chronic recurrent infection.
(c) All the vaginal commensal organisms, staphylococci, streptococci, coliforms, chlamydia,
gonococcus or tuberculosis.
(d) The bowel (large and small) related to adhesions, the ureter, or bladder.

56 **(a)** Probably not, but granuloma inguinale or tropical bubo are possibilities.
(b) The vulva, vagina, or uterus. It is unlikely to be a lymphoma, trophoblastic disease, or
melanoma
(c) The femoral and inguinal nodes, but this does depend on the frozen section of the biopsy.
(d) The presence of a swelling or lump rather than pain.

57 **(a)** CIN II or CIN III.
(b) There is a coarse punctate pattern suggestive of a carcinoma-in-situ.
(c) It could be treated while awaiting the result of a punch biopsy from the abnormal area.
(d) CIN III.

58 **(a)** Diabetes mellitus.
(b) Glucose tolerance test (GTT).
(c) Shoulder dystocia.
(d) Yes, there is a higher incidence of fetal abnormality in association with maternal diabetes.

59 **(a)** No, because it indicates at least a bicornuate uterus.
(b) Breech or transverse lie.
(c) Third-stage problems.
(d) The uterine shape in the later weeks of pregnancy, particularly with a contraction, should have revealed a bicornuate shape on inspection or palpation.

60 **(a)** Vulval biopsy.
(b) In the preparation of the patient there has been trauma to the skin by swabbing, which resulted in bleeding.
(c) Lichen sclerosus, VIN II or VIN III.
(d) There should be symptomatic relief in the absence of malignant change. Removal of the abnormal area is likely to be followed by a recurrence after a period of time.

61 **(a)** Double uterus with some dye leaking into the vagina and dye in both fallopian tubes and possible spill of dye on both sides.
(b) Vaginal septum and renal abnormality (see 51).
(c) If there was no contraindication then the combined oral contraceptive pill could be tried as it is usually effective in these cases.
(d) There may be a threat to abort or actual abortion, antepartum hemorrhage (APH), or premature labor (there is likely to be decidual bleeding intermittently from the nonpregnant uterus).

62 **(a)** Prinicipally, 'These may seriously damage your health' with variations.
(b) Smoking affects placental function and can produce a 'small-for-dates' baby.
(c) The breakdown products of tobacco are excreted in cervical mucus and the sexual practises of smokers are different.
(d) Epidemiological studies suggests that the risks of taking the combined oral contraceptive pill are of the order of smoking one-third of a cigarette for 3 weeks out of 4.

63 **(a)** No. There are white and pigmented areas.
(b) No, but there are flat plaques present.
(c) No, but that does not exclude the possibility of carcinoma being present.
(d) **(ii)** wide excision of abnormal area.

64 **(a)** Not possible. Three clips on cords are visible, a structure on the lower right side could be another cord.
(b) Induction of ovulation and assisted reproduction.
(c) Anemia, abortion, APH, pre-eclampsia, premature labor, and an increase of the usual pregnancy symptoms.
(d) Yes, this applies to all multiple pregnancies, including twin pregnancy.

65 **(a)** It would appear that there is a subumbilical vertical scar, which reaches one-third of the distance from the symphysis pubis to the umbilicus and a right paramedian incision, which commences from the upper part of the midline incision that extends upwards beyond the

umbilicus. There may be a Cesarean section scar or minor gynecological operation (midline scar) and a laparotomy, possibly for ovarian carcinoma. There may also be an appendicectomy scar or drain site on the RIF.
(b) Possibly a secondary nodule of tumor.
(c) It would depend on whether the patient has had chemotherapy before, but some form of chemotherapy would be appropriate.
(d) Overall poor, particularly with a proven ovarian adenocarcinoma.

66 **(a)** Ruptured horn of a bicornuate uterus.
(b) The rupture probably occurred at 12–14 weeks rather than 6–8 weeks.
(c) The patient should be seen as soon as the pregnancy is confirmed to check if it is intrauterine and if there are any unusual symptoms.
(d) Delivery should be by Cesarean section as there would be a risk of uterine rupture.

67 **(a)** Carcinoma of the clitoris.
(b) To the femoral and inguinal nodes plus obturator and around the internal iliac vessels, particularly the veins.
(c) Modified radical vulvectomy and removal of all appropriate lymph nodes.
(d) At least half.

68 **(a)** Hydrocolpos behind an imperforate hymen.
(b) Incise the membrane and allow spontaneous drainage.
(c) Infection.
(d) No.

69 **(a)** No, there is a discolored area at the right fornix.
(b) Possibly endometriosis.
(c) Excise it and, if appropriate, give danazol or a combined oral contraceptive for 3–6 months.
(d) There is risk to the bladder and ureter.

70 **(a)** Vulval varicosities.
(b) Yes.
(c) During the later part of pregnancy.
(d) In pregnancy, advise rest. If the patient is not pregnant, they could be injected or ligated.

71 **(a)** Screening for AFP levels and ultrasound, plus increased use of legal abortion criteria.
(b) Yes.
(c) Yes, multivitamin therapy, particularly folic acid for at least 3 months prior to conception.
(d) About 1:100 if no previous central nervous system (CNS) abnormalities.

72 **(a)** No, it is an endocervical polyp.
(b) Excise it.
(c) The base is incompletely excised.
(d) Yes.

73 **(a)** The uterus, tube, and a cyst.
(b) If the other ovary is normal, remove the cyst, i.e. oophorectomy or salpingo-oophorectomy.

(c) Give danazol for 6–8 months.
(d) Oophorectomy or salpingo-oophorectomy and regular follow-up.

74 **(a)** A retention cyst of an endocervical gland.
(b) Either by blockage of the opening with a plug of mucus or by squamous metaplasia of the epithelium at the entrance of the gland to occlude the opening.
(c) It would be excised and the base treated by diathermy.
(d) Multiple.

75 **(a)** The appearance suggests it has been present for a long time.
(b) Vaginal hysterectomy and repair.
(c) An enterocele.
(d) Insertion of a ring pessary; sometimes a shelf pessary may be required.

76 **(a)** A sebaceous cyst in perineum.
(b) Pain or dyspareunia.
(c) Excision.
(d) No.

77 **(a)** 46XY or a mosaicism.
(b) There is a risk of the gonads becoming malignant.
(c) An androblastoma.
(d) Not to any great extent.

78 **(a)** It was more likely to be dead.
(b) With multiple pregnancy or premature deliveries.
(c) Foot and hand with breech presentation.
(d) Assess when admitted in labor with ultrasound and decide whether to have a Cesarean section or vaginal delivery.

79 **(a)** There is an increase in the melanocyte activity.
(b) With the combined oral contraceptive pill in some women.
(c) Abdomen linea nigra, neck, breasts, vulva, and nevi may become more pigmented.
(d) Yes.

80 **(a)** Intertrigo podicis.
(b) Yes.
(c) Yes.
(d) Yes.

81 **(a)** Invasive carcinoma of the cervix.
(b) Squamous cell carcinoma and the degree of differentiation and also whether there is any evidence of vascular involvement.
(c) With an obvious carcinoma Stage IB or more advanced lesion it is not helpful, as a biopsy can be taken without the need for colposcopy. It is mainly done for learning/teaching purposes.
(d) About 30%.

Self-assessment picture tests
Obstetrics and Gynecology

82 **(a)** A fibroid uterus.
(b) A complaint of infertility.
(c) Yes, because of the distorted shape of the uterine cavity. They are likely to be multiple leiomyomata.
(d) Abortion, malpresentation, red degeneration of the leiomyomata, problems in labor, and postpartum hemorrhage.

83 **(a)** Benign.
(b) Remove the base of the tumor and reconstitute the cervix.
(c) Yes, the cervix reaches the introitus with traction on the tumor.
(d) A sensation of something in the vagina or a lump coming out of the vagina.

84 **(a)** Torsion of an ovary or a parovarian cyst.
(b) The histology of the tumor, type, and differentiation.
(c) At this age, fertility and retention of the uterus is likely to be a factor, so it may be appropriate to arrange for a course of chemotherapy.
(d) AFP, HCG and/or CA 125.

85 **(a)** Occipitoposterior presentation and/or delay.
(b) There should be a reasonable chance of success, uterine contractions present, membranes ruptured, preferably an empty bladder and rectum, and the cervix preferably fully dilated, but this is not essential.
(c) No, but one is often performed when there is a posterior presentation.
(d) It can be used when the cervix is not fully dilated.

86 **(a)** Either because of vulval soreness or irritation, or the mother considered that her daughter was not normal.
(b) A bland cream or even local estrogen cream after separation of the fused labia.
(c) No, but it does occur.
(d) No, because the labia are fused and look slightly edematous.

87 **(a)** Carcinoma of the vulva with an obvious node on the left side. This was, however, a melanoma.
(b) It is the proposed area of excision.
(c) Almost certainly a graft would be required.
(d) It would be appropriate if technically easy because the lump approaching the iliac crest would suggest that the glands may well be involved.

88 **(a)** This is the hand of a woman with systemic lupus erythematosus (SLE).
(b) There is a high risk of abortion, perinatal loss, pre-eclampsia, hypertension in pregnancy, antepartum hemorrhage, disseminated intravascular coagulation (DIC), and thromboembolism.
(c) Yes. Antinuclear antibodies (ANA) are present in 99% of patients who have the disease and an assay for anti-DNA antibodies should be done if the ANA test is positive as the antibodies are believed to play a causal role in the syndrome of neonatal lupus.
(d) Fetal loss is at least double that of the general population. Exacerbation of the SLE occurs in 30–50% of pregnant women.

89 **(a)** Vesicovaginal fistula.
(b) Operative trauma during vaginal delivery, a vaginal gynecological operation, or hysterectomy.
(c) Good at first operation, provided that the surgeon is experienced.
(d) Deliver by Cesarean section.

90 **(a)** Carcinoma (probably adenocarcinoma).
(b) Carcinoma of the endometrium or cervix, rather than a primary vaginal carcinoma.
(c) With radiotherapy.
(d) An anterior exenteration.

91 **(a)** Female circumcision.
(b) Sudan and Somalia.
(c) Tears at the time of delivery, and hemorrhage.
(d) No, it is illegal.

92 **(a)** Cone biopsy of the cervix with anterior and posterior Sturmdorf's sutures.
(b) Secondary hemorrhage, incompetent or stenosed cervix in any future pregnancy.
(c) Loop diathermy excision, laser conization, or using the cold coagulation technique.
(d) CIN III or microinvasive carcinoma of the cervix or, if the CIN III lesion on the cervix extends into the canal and cannot be totally visualized, by colposcopy.

93 **(a)** Lichen sclerosus.
(b) It not infrequently resolves spontaneously.
(c) Topical steroids.
(d) 3–4%.

94 **(a)** A previous vulvectomy.
(b) Hemorrhoid.
(c) Hemorrhoidectomy (excision of the hemorrhoid).
(d) No.

95 **(a)** Normal squamous cells.
(b) Mature and immature cells (squamous metaplasia).
(c) Cervix (cervical smear).
(d) If the ratio of the size of the nucleus to cytoplasm increased and there was considerable irregularity of the nuclei.

96 **(a)** Round ligaments.
(b) Endometriosis.
(c) The ovarian vessels.
(d) Just below the ovarian vessels.

97 **(a)** The peak incidence in 1968 was between 45 and 54 but in 1979 there is a suggestion of two peaks, one at 30–40 and another at 55–65.
(b) Yes.
(c) Possibly more cases were diagnosed with preinvasive disease (CIN) in 1979 or the incidence of the disease was falling.
(d) No, because the total population is unknown and only the rate per 100,000 is given.

98 **(a)** An enlarged abdominal wall with a multiloculated cyst.
(b) Yes.
(c) Because it is multiloculated and there are solid areas present.
(d) Serous cystadenocarcinoma.

99 **(a)** Carcinoma.
(b) Papillary hidradenoma.
(c) Local excision.
(d) A sweat gland.

100 **(a)** Carcinoma of the cervix.
(b) No, but the incidence of pelvic and para-aortic node involvement would be expected to be higher.
(c) No, postoperative radiotherapy would be required.
(d) Postcoital and/or intermenstrual bleeding and offensive vaginal discharge.

101 **(a)** An abnormal posterior lip of cervix with abnormal vasculature and bleeding.
(b) A carcinoma of the cervix.
(c) If there is no evidence of a lesion other than on the posterior lip of the cervix then a radical hysterectomy would be recommended, i.e. if Stage IB and possibly IIA. If IIB or greater then radiotherapy is preferable. If imaging techniques reveal pelvic wall lymph node involvement, then radiotherapy is indicated.
(d) Yes, it may be possible to conserve the ovaries in a younger woman if she has surgery for Stage IB and there is no lymph node spread.

102 **(a)** Monilial vulvovaginitis.
(b) The pH is usually 4.5 or lower.
(c) Broad-spectrum antibiotics, diabetes mellitus, pregnancy, high-dose oral contraceptives, and altered host immunity (e.g. immunosuppressive drugs or AIDS). There may be local factors, e.g. increased vaginal warmth, increased vaginal moisture, and tight/occlusive clothing.
(d) Topical creams or pessaries that contain polyenes or imidazoles, e.g. nystatin, clotrimazole, or miconazole.

103 **(a)** It is positive (abnormal).
(b) There is an increased risk of Down's syndrome
(c) 1:90.
(d) 1:880. An ultrasound should be arranged to confirm the gestational age. A screen-positive result indicates an increased risk of having a pregnancy with Down's syndrome or a neural tube defect.

104 **(a)** In this case a short history of vaginal bleeding (1 month), abdominal distension (1 week), and abdominal pain (4 days).
(b) A mixed mesodermal tumor of the tube. It was not the more common emergency of ectopic pregnancy. The embryonic type is associated with development defects. Other, less common, causes of this rare tumor are irradiation of the endometrium and abnormal stimulation with estrogen.
(c) Abdominal hysterectomy and bilateral salpingo-oophorectomy (TAH & BSO), radiotherapy and, chemotherapy.
(d) 1–2% of all sarcomas.

105 **(a)** CA 125 is a high molecular weight glycoprotein antigenic determinant recognized by the murine glycoprotein OC 125.
(b) In ovarian carcinoma, endometriosis, and diverticular disease.
(c) Perform a pelvic ultrasound, laparoscopy, and surgery for removal of ovarian cyst.
(d) Residual ovarian cancer if ovarian tumor found at operation.

106 **(a)** A cardiotocograph in labor.
(b) **(i)** Regular contractions of the uterus; **(ii)** type 2 dips, i.e. decelerations lasting after the uterine contractions; and **(iii)** a slight rise in the fetal heart rate after the dips, suggesting the fetus has reserves and is able to compensate for possible anoxia.
(c) Assess the mother, perform a vaginal examination, and take a fetal blood sample. Depending on the findings, it may be necessary to deliver the fetus.
(d) Trauma to the fetus, bleeding, and it may lead to excessive intervention.

107 **(a)** **(1)** Hinkson Edwards caudal needle, **(2)** flanged Tuohy needle, **(3)** epidural needle, **(4)** pudendal block needle, **(5)** Cooper's paracervical block needle.
(b) Consent must be obtained. Set up an intravenous infusion and preload the maternal circulation with 1 litre of Hartmann's solution as blood may pool in the lower limb veins.
(c) It is good for simple lift-out forceps, but needs perineal infiltration and it does not give adequate analgesia for a rotational forceps.
(d) Intravenous and intra-arterial injection. Local anesthetic may be absorbed and enter the fetal circulation.

108 **(a)** Clips for female sterilization. **(1)** Hulka, **(2)** Filshie, and **(3)** later modification Filshie.
(b) 1 in 500–1000 procedures.
(c) Clips not properly applied to the tube so as to occlude the fallopian tube lumen. They may be applied to the round ligament in error. Occasionally they can cut through the tube allowing an open end for the spermatozoa to pass up and the ovum to pass down (N.B. increased risk of ectopic pregnancy).
(d) Laparoscopy, although they can be applied at laparotomy.

109 **(a)** **(1)** Kjelland's forceps, **(2)** Neville Barnes axis traction forceps, **(3)** Wrigley's forceps.
(b) To allow for a rotation and forceps delivery and to be able to correct asynclitism.
(c) Axis traction allows a very strong pull to be exerted, but the arrow on the axis traction handle means that the pull can be exerted in the axis of the pelvis.
(d) So that not too much pull can be exerted at delivery. By having a short handle this instrument can easily be used for the after-coming head of the breech or used at a Cesarean section delivery.

110 **(a)** (1) Blunt curette, (2) sharp curette, and (3) flushing curette.
(b) Perforation. The blunt curette presents a fine end and, therefore, is more likely to perforate. The sharp curette presents a wider end and perforation is, therefore, less likely.
(c) Hysteroscopy.
(d) Hysteroscopy allows a visually guided biopsy to be taken; therefore, a more accurate diagnosis is made.

111, 112
(a) The lateral view cystogram (111) and IVU (112) show the presence of radiocontrast in the vagina. This confirms that there is a vesicovaginal fistula (VVF). Bladder and ureteric injuries

of this type occur in approximately 0.3–0.5% of all hysterectomies.

(b) True (continuous) incontinence. Although this may occur immediately, it is often delayed until after the patient has been discharged. There may be urinary infection and upper urinary tract sepsis if ureteric drainage is impaired in any way.

(c) If a VVF is suspected, intravenous pyelography followed by a cystoscopy, EUA and a 'three swab' test should be performed. A urine sample should also be sent for culture.

(d) Having defined the anatomical problem and treated any urinary tract infection, the fistula should be closed surgically. This may be done abdominally, or vaginally, or combined. Fistulas of this type should be corrected by gynecologists or urologists with experience in fistula surgery.

113 (a) Autosomal dominant inheritance.
(b) No, because male-to-male transmission.
(c) (i) and **(ii)** Yes: **(iii)** and **(iv)** No.
(d) A's children 1 in 2 risk: B's children no risk.

114 (a) Vulval hematoma.
(b) Falling across a bicycle crossbar or gymnastic bar or, as in this case, being kicked by a horse.
(c) Ice packs and/or incise and drain the blood, ligating or diathermy any bleeding points.
(d) Infection and nerve injury can occur with horse kick injuries.

115 (a) Genetic, physiological, adrenal causes, ovarian causes, sexual abnormalities, iatrogenic or other miscellaneous causes, including acromegaly. It was associated with an adrenal tumor.
(b) Hormone investigations include testosterone, androstenedione, dehydroepiandrosterone and its sulfate, FSH, LH, and thyroid stimulating hormone (TSH), cortisol levels and urinary ketosteroids. Perform ultrasound of ovaries and adrenal glands and CT or MRI scans if any doubt.
(c) Pathological.
(d) Cushing's syndrome due to adrenocortical hyperplasia or adrenal tumors (benign or malignant). Androgen production from a tumor is unlikely to be suppressed by dexamethasone, as in this case, where there was a benign adrenal tumor.

116 (a) A male patient with trisomy 21.
(b) Yes.
(c) Yes, particularly affecting the heart, gastrointestinal tract, eye, and ear.
(d) By maternal AFP screening, triple test screening, amniocentesis, and cell culture.

117 (a) Bilateral hydrosalpinges.
(b) Pelvic infection, possibly due to gonococcal or chlamydial infection. Alternatively, it may be due to nonspecific organisms, such as *Bacteroides, E. coli,* mycoplasma or viruses.
(c) Dysmenorrhea, menorrhagia, dyspareunia, backache, or lower abdominal pain.
(d) Not usually. Removal of the tubes and in-vitro fertilization (IVF) techniques offer the best chance of achieving a pregnancy.

118 (a) Dyspareunia or inability to have intercourse,
(b) Incise the tissue defined by the probe and reconstruct the vaginal introitus.
(c) It could be developmental, but in fact this was caused by some chemical used to induce an abortion.
(d) Yes, unless there is other damage to the genital tract.

119 **(a)** Female circumcision.
(b) Vaginal delivery will be associated with vaginal tears.
(c) Not usually.
(d) No, it is cultural and banned in most countries.

120 **(a)** Urethral caruncle or carcinoma (but rare).
(b) Postmenopausal.
(c) It may improve with local estrogen cream, but it is usual to excise it after carrying out a cystoscopy.
(d) It is a benign growth covered by transitional epithelium and may contain some nerve fibres.

121 **(a)** *Trichomonas vaginalis.*
(b) It is a flagellated protozoon and a strict anaerobe.
(c) Vaginal discharge and irritation. There is a strawberry red appearance in the vagina. There is a greenish discharge with bubbles present and sometimes a fishy odor.
(d) Metronidazole.

122 **(a)** An abnormal vascular pattern with single and coiled capillaries.
(b) Yes.
(c) Yes.
(d) Not known precisely, but studies suggest that about 15% if aged over 35 and 30–40% if under 35 years of age.

123 **(a)** The middle one.
(b) The one to the right.
(c) The left one.
(d) Approximately 95% (19 in 20).

124, 125
(a) Yes, the soft tissue swelling in the neck (nuchal fold).
(b) Yes.
(c) Yes.
(d) The ear.

126 **(a)** Poor iodine take-up over the whole of the cervix.
(b) It is one option.
(c) If endocervical smears were normal.
(d) Yes, a proportion of patients will develop VAIN III and possibly neoplasia.

127, 128
(a) Bilateral internal iliac adenopathy.
(b) No.
(c) Tumor recurrence in the posterior vaginal vault and infiltration of the left paracolpos soft tissue; bilateral internal iliac adenopathy and probable rectal infiltration.
(d) Radiotherapy, because posterior or total exenteration is unlikely to have long-term success because of pelvic node involvement.

129–131

(a) A large bulky tumor arising from the cervix, displacing the vaginal vault posteriorly, and invading the upper third of the vagina.

(b) There is a tumor arising from the cervix and a large left pelvic sidewall node.

(c) There is extensive stranding within the parametrial soft tissues, indicating infiltration.

(d) Radical radiotherapy centrally and to the pelvic sidewalls and to the lower part of the para-aortic nodes.

132, 133

(a) There is a collection of fluid within the posterior fornix and uterus.

(b) There is a definite collection of fluid within the posterior fornix.

(c) A collection of fluid, possibly infected, in the upper vagina and uterus.

(d) Antibiotic therapy to cover EUA and drainage of the vagina and dilatation of the cervix. Send material for culture and histology if any tissue is removed. That is often all that is necessary but, sometimes, a hysterectomy is indicated; this should be carried out only by surgeons familiar with operating on irradiated tissue.

134, 135

(a) There is a mixed solid/cystic mass in the right adnexal region. There is a large volume of ascites anteriorly.

(b) The upper abdomen reveals ascites and cystic metastases in the liver.

(c) Ovarian carcinoma, probably a serous cystadenocarcinoma.

(d) TAH & BSO, omentectomy and chemotherapy. It would not be justified to remove the multiple liver metastases. The prognosis is poor and the survival time is likely to be only of the order of 18–20 months.

136 (a) It demonstrates a large, predominantly right-sided, cystic mass, which is intimately related to adjacent bowel loops resulting in a fistula (note the presence of air within the mass).

(b) A metastatic deposit from a primary carcinoma of the ovary.

(c) A laparotomy.

(d) Palliative.

137–139

(a) There is a large cystic/solid mass in the central pelvis, with displacement of the uterus and rectum.

(b) A large central pelvic mass adherent to the sigmoid colon and rectum.

(c) Subsquent histology proved it to be a melanoma.

(d) No, palliative chemotherapy only.

140, 141

(a) The cord on the placenta on the left side suggests a previously viable cord compared with the other cord. Membranes are on one placenta. There may be some small nodules on the lower part of the left placenta.

(b) They represent amniotic nodosum.

(c) They are often associated with oligohydramnios.

(d) Intrauterine death and renal agenesis.

142 (a) Pedunculated papilloma or fibroma.

(b) The labia majora.

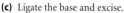
(c) Ligate the base and excise.
(d) Not obviously, but the base looks slightly atrophic.

143 (a) A spill of dye in the pelvis and an enlarged uterus with the possibility of polyps in the uterus.
(b) Hysteroscopy.
(c) Most probably an abortion.
(d) It cannot be stated with certainty, but there is a 40–50% possibility of improving her chances.

144 (a) Cervical cancer.
(b) More screening, better recall, and earlier diagnosis and treatment.
(c) Ovarian cancer.
(d) No, despite better chemotherapeutic agents.

145 (a) Yes.
(b) No.
(c) Advantage: less vascular. Disadvantage: increased risk of extension to the sphincter ani.
(d) About 40%.

146 (a) A uterus with either a rudimentary horn or a bicornuate uterus; the former was diagnosed.
(b) Removal of the rudimentary horn.
(c) If conserved, it will be detached from the uterus.
(d) Apart from cosmetic factors (smaller scars) and much quicker postoperative recovery, laparoscopic procedures are said to result in far fewer adhesions postoperatively. It is not an easy operation whichever route is chosen (abdominally with modified type of Strassman procedure) and should be done only by surgeons familiar with the appropriate techniques.

147 (a) Ovarian cyst.
(b) Fibroid uterus.
(c) Normal right adnexa.
(d) Normal appendix.

148 (a) Rollerball endometrial ablation.
(b) Menorrhagia.
(c) It avoids a hysterectomy in the majority of cases and it can be performed as day case or an overnight stay.
(d) Inexperience of the operator.

149 (a) Multiple pregnancy is more common and, therefore, more likely.
(b) Pass a nasogastric tube to exclude esophageal atresia.
(c) In all probability by repeat Cesarean section.
(d) Malignant.

150 (a) No
(b) CIN III. Please refer for colposcopy.
(c) Cervical screening is for preinvasive disease and breast screening is for early stage invasive disease.
(d) Breast screening (per person) is 10 times as expensive as cervical screening.

MCQ Answers

True answers only:

151 ABD	**166** BD	**181** C	**196** ACDE
152 BC	**167** ACD	**182** ABE	**197** CDE
153 AE	**168** CDE	**183** C	**198** ABC
154 AC	**169** D	**184** D	**199** ABE
155 BCE	**170** CDE	**185** ACE	**200** ABC
156 CDE	**171** BD	**186** AD	**201** AD
157 ABCD	**172** BDE	**187** AE	**202** AE
158 BDE	**173** BCDE	**188** AD	**203** AB
159 CDE	**174** ACD	**189** AC	**204** CDE
160 CD	**175** ACD	**190** ACE	**205** ABE
161 ABDE	**176** AC	**191** CD	**206** DE
162 CE	**177** BCD	**192** A	**207** ABC
163 ABE	**178** D	**193** BCD	**208** ABE
164 DE	**179** ABCD	**194** DE	**209** BDE
165 CE	**180** AD	**195** AC	**210** BD

Note from author:
It should be appreciated that with clinical multiple choice questions there may be
exceptions to an individual statement or question posed. The reader may disagree with
our opinion regarding the answers but the real educational exercise is finding the truth.
That is what makes the practice of medicine an art as well as a science.

ICH Answers

Case 211

1. **(a)** Twins. Advise the mother that she should be seen regularly.
   (b) The risks are: premature labor (give steroids from 26 weeks' gestation?); antepartum hemorrhage; intra-uterine growth retardation (regular ultrasound scans necessary); anemia (give supplementary iron and folic acid); pre-eclampsia (early detection as seen regularly); and fetal abnormality about one to three times greater than singleton pregnancy

2. The normal range for AFP included 2.5 multiples of the medium (MoM). The AFP is raised but within normal limits for a twin pregnancy. There is, therefore, no need to repeat the test.

3. The mother should be told that one fetus has disappeared, but the other fetus appears to be growing normally and is compatible with dates. Death of one fetus is said to occur in 1–7% of multiple pregnancies.

4. The mother was approaching term and had had a twin pregnancy; one of the fetuses had died in utero. It is unknown if it is a uniovular or binovular twin pregnancy. The consultant considered there was an increased risk for the remaining fetus and there was a risk of disseminated intravascular coagulation (DIC). Also, vaginal findings indicated favorable features for induction (Bishop score).

5. Gradually increase the oxytocin as for agreed hospital protocol, which varies from hospital to hospital. When good uterine contractions are present and labor established then maintain dosage or reduce. Review CTG regularly and carry out 3–4 hourly vaginal examinations to assess progress. The midwife to inform you if there are any problems (so that you can assess the situation personally) and when the mother is fully dilated. Otherwise see the mother on routine labor ward rounds.

6. The CTG shows poor variability after there had been good beat-to-beat variations. It was decided to continue observations and review in 2 hours.

7. **(a)** Allow vaginal delivery but obligatory episiotomy. If there is any deviation from normal, the medical staff to be contacted.
   (b) The incidence is about 1:500.
   (c) A persistent mentoposterior presentation cannot be delivered vaginally but, if good uterine action occurs, the chin may rotate through the transverse position to become mentoanterior. If it does not then Cesarean delivery will be necessary.

8. A fetus papyraceous (FP) itself could have abnormalities, in keeping with a higher incidence of fetal abnormalities in multiple pregnancies. The incidence of FP is about 1:1000–1500.

9. The 'caput' forms over the face and it can be contused and bruised, and sucking, initially, may be difficult. Reassure the mother as it usually resolves in 24–48 hours.

Case 212

1. The color should change to orange.

2. **(a)** It is a footling breech. The classification is based on the attitude of the fetal legs and whether the hip or knee joints are flexed or extended. The complete breech has both joints flexed. The incomplete breech occurs when there is extension of both hip and knee joints to give a footling (single or double) presentation; when the hip joint is flexed and the knee joint extended there is a frank breech, which is more common at full term because the splint-like effect of the extended legs prevents spontaneous rotation of the breech in the later weeks of pregnancy (see 212h).
    (b) Prolapse of the umbilical cord following the membranes rupturing.

3. **(a)** To avoid silent gastric regurgitation (Mendelson's syndrome); if it does occur then aspiration of the contents into the lungs will be more alkaline than acid.
    (b) H_2-agonists (receptor blockers), e.g. ranitidine, are now preferred to antacids.

4. **(a)** Cricoid pressure is applied to avoid regurgitation after administration of anesthetic agents and muscle relaxants, prior to endotracheal intubation.
    (b) Aspiration of gastric contents, hypoxia due to problems with intubation, or misplaced tracheal intubation.

5. **(a)** It is less vascular and it heals better. There is both less blood loss and risk of infection.
    (b) Lower segment Cesarean section scars rarely rupture (less than 0.25%), but if they do it is likely to be during labor. Classical Cesarean section scars may rupture (3–4%) late in pregnancy as well as in labor.
    (c) Transverse lie with back downwards and unapproachable lower segment due to fibroids or placenta praevia.

6. **(a)** Yes, it is now accepted practise but it varies (all or selected cases) from unit to unit.
    (b) The antibiotic(s) should cover the likely aerobic and anaerobic organisms associated with pelvic infection. Metronidazole and cefuroxime should be given, or erythromycin if the mother is penicillin sensitive. Another alternative is amoxicillin alone.

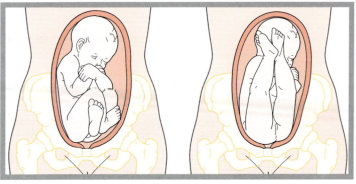

← **212h**

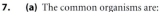

7. **(a)** The common organisms are:
   (i) aerobic streptococci, anaerobic Gram-positive cocci, and
   (ii) aerobic (e.g. *E. coli*) and an aerobic Gram-negative bacilli (e.g. *Bacteroides*).
   (b) Concurrent wound infection and resistant micro-organisms.
   (c) Because the reason for the Cesarean section was a malpresentation then, provided that the pelvis is adequate and the presentation and size of the fetus reasonable, a vaginal delivery is likely.

Case 213

1. **(a)** Ovulatory bleeding midcycle is one cause, but intermenstrual bleeding is usually associated with bleeding of variable quantity and occurring at any time in the menstrual cycle. Common causes are fibroids and endometrial, endocervica,l or cervical polyps, which are usually benign in a woman aged 42 years. Occasionally, intermenstrual bleeding can be due to a chronic endometritis or be iatrogenic, related to hormonal preparations.
   (b) The role of dilatation and curettage, particularly in the investigation of menorrhagia, has been criticized because a significant proportion of lesions are missed. It has been suggested that hysteroscopy, as a day case or an outpatient, to allow the inside of the uterus to be inspected, and the newer outpatient endometrial sampling methods, are more appropriate and achieve a more accurate diagnosis.

2. **(a)** There are the potential complications of the distending media, including fluid overload, embolism, and anaphylaxis. Surgical risks include uterine perforation, infection, and bleeding.
   (b) There are few. Acute pelvic infections, menstruation, and pregnancy are the obvious ones, but others are related to the patient's fitness for a general anesthetic.

3. Benign. The polyp is mainly composed of congested and focally inflamed stroma: note the thick-walled blood vessels.

4. A detailed sexual history should be taken and you should determine if the woman is still having, and wishes to continue to have, intercourse.

5. **(a)** William Edward Fothergill was a Manchester gynecologist whose name is associated with Donald's in relation to the surgical treatment of prolapse. Fothergill's points are related to the urethral meatus and placing clamps to mark the position of the cardinal ligaments lateral to the cervix. The points are so called because Fothergill advocated exposure of the cardinal ligaments to facilitate their approximation in front of the cervix in a Manchester repair operation. The principle of exposing, and repositioning, the cardinal ligaments is important, the points are not.
   (b) Local infiltration is used to separate the tissue layers prior to the removal of the excess vaginal epithelium. If dilute solutions of epinephrine are used, the amount of local bleeding is reduced.

6. Some gynecologists use suprapubic catheters, some leave Foley catheters in overnight or for 24 hours, and others do not catheterize unless the patient cannot pass urine postoperatively.

7. Variable, but incidence can be as high as 5%.

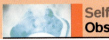
8. There is an increasing tendency to use intraoperative antibiotics for major operations, especially if catheters are likely to be left in situ.

Case 214

1. History: In Mrs A's history it is important to identify any irregularity of the menstrual cycle as this may indicate an ovulation problem. Any intermenstrual or post coital bleeding should be noted. The obstetric history, if any, should detail any antenatal or postnatal problems. The medical history should cover ongoing systemic illnesses, any previous gynecological problems, in particular ectopic pregnancy and suspected or proven pelvic infection, and record any abdominal surgery. With regard to her partner, the history should include details of any children he may have fathered or any previous illnesses. It is particularly important to obtain information about any pyrexial illnesses in the preceding 6 months as this can lower sperm count significantly. Check if there is any history of orchitis, epididymitis, torsion or maldescent of the testes, or varicocele. Details of any treatment, including at what age any surgery was performed, are required. History of any sexually transmitted diseases (STD) should be noted. Social factors of relevance are smoking and alcohol, as both nicotine and alcohol can affect sperm counts and function. The sexual history of both partners should cover problems of dyspareunia, erection or ejaculation. It is also important to ascertain whether the couple are aware of, and use, the fertile period, and an estimate of coital frequency should be obtained.

2. Examination of Mrs A should be appropriate to detect any signs of underlying endocrine disorder, e.g. hirsutism, galactorrhea, and other manifestations of endocrine disease. The height and weight have already been noted and, by themselves, do not reflect an ovulatory problem. An abdominal and pelvic examination are necessary to detect any uterine abnormality or any adnexal pathology. Examination of the partner is required to detect any urogenital abnormality not revealed by the history. Testicular size and volume should be noted and also any varicocele, epididymal thickening, or scrotal swelling.

3. For Mrs A, an irregular infrequent cycle, oligomenorrhea (cycle greater than 42 days, but less than 6 months), amenorrhea (of at least 6 months), previous ectopic pregnancy, history of pelvic infection or STD, abdominal surgery, or any significant abnormality on physical examination. For her partner, a history of testicular maldescent, previous genital pathology, including orchitis and varicocele or STD, any urogenital surgery, and any abnormality on physical examination.

4. Yes, the results are acceptable.

5. The minor uterine abnormality (214a) with slight spill of dye. The double uterine cavity (214b) may be associated with problems in pregnancy and fetal loss. The loculation of the dye (214c) suggests previous infection and also may be associated with an ectopic pregnancy if conception occurs.

6. 214d indicates a very marked response on the first course of clomiphene (mild overstimulation) and no ovulation with the second course. 214e demonstrates ovulation and levels of estrogen and progesterone indicating pregnancy. It should be noted that there is variable response in the three cycles to an identical dose of clomiphene.

7. 214f shows no response to clomiphene, despite supplementing the latter part of the cycle with progesterone. In comparison, in 214g, with a small dose of follicle stimulating hormone (FSH) and human chorionic gonadotrophin (HCG), conception and pregnancy resulted. This is a satisfactory result in a case of unexplained subfertility.

8. In the woman who had radiotherapy to the pituitary gland, 214i shows no response initially to FSH but the second course, with an increased dose of FSH plus HCG, indicates ovulation and the first menstrual period for 10 years. 214i shows no response with an identical dose of FSH and HCG compared with the second course shown in 214h. As a result of increasing the dosage of FSH to seven ampoules on days 1, 3, and 5, followed by HCG, conception occurred and resulted in the successful delivery of a child by Cesarean section at 38 weeks' gestation. There is a very individual response to FSH and HCG. This pattern would be similar to that of women who now have their pituitary gonadotrophic function temporarily stopped by 'downregulation therapy' and then given FSH and HCG.

Case 215

1. The most likely diagnosis for Mrs M is Paget's disease; Mrs C has lichen sclerosus, and Ms F has hyperplasia of the squamous epithelium.

2. The appropriate treatment for Mrs M would be (b).
    The most appropriate treatment and management for Mrs C would be (c).
    The treatment option for Ms F is (a).

3. Paget's disease of the vulva, unlike Paget's disease of the breast, is usually an adenocarcinoma-in-situ. In about 30% of cases there is an underlying invasive tumor, which may be in the adjacent vulval area, the anal canal, or the urinary tract. Rarely, the adenocarcinoma-in-situ may progress to invasive carcinoma.

4. If a woman with Paget's disease of the vulva develops a 'lump', the possibility of a primary or secondary vulva carcinoma should always be excluded. A biopsy of the 'lump' is essential and, if malignant, appropriate radical treatment carried out.

5. The development of epithelial hyperplasia in a woman with lichen sclerosus is an indication for repeat biopsy. Women with epithelial hyperplasia and lichen sclerosus are those who are at risk of developing squamous carcinoma. If a carcinoma is present, radical treatment is necessary. If not, then regular and continuous observation with conservative treatment is appropriate. Sometimes, a simple vulvectomy may be required to obtain relief for a period of time, but it is never curative.

6. The borderline nuclear changes in Ms F's smear may be indicative of human papilloma virus (HPV) infection of the cervix. The appearance of the vulva is also consistent with HPV-associated vulval intraepithelial neoplasiam (VIN), probably HPV Type 16. The warts that developed in her teens may not have been associated with an oncogenic HPV type.

7. The development of a lump in a patient with VIN may indicate the development of invasive carcinoma. Urgent biopsy is mandatory.

8. The accepted treatment until the mid-1970s and early-1980s was radical vulvectomy, when a large excess of skin was removed, particularly over the mons pubis. The current treatment involves bilateral groin incisions to remove the superficial and deep femoral and inguinal lymph nodes, and a simple vulvectomy or an adequate excision at the site of the carcinoma. This results in far lower morbidity, a shorter stay in hospital, and a similar cure rate. The most appropriate treatment for carcinoma of the anus is radiotherapy, with or without surgery. Depending on the size of the lesion, preoperative radiotherapy followed by surgery may be indicated. Obviously, if the anal sphincter is going to be impaired, then a colostomy may be required, either temporary or permanent (with or without an abdominoperineal excision of the rectum).

Case 216

1. The precise reason for the association of fibroids and subfertility is unknown. However, the fibroid was unlikely to be a direct factor. There could be a male factor because no details are given or had been requested.

2. All too often they are considered to be a factor but, in this case, the menstrual cycle was probably the major factor, in combination with anovulation.

3. No, not without full investigation of other causes for the couple's inability to conceive in 2 years. Because ovulation was confirmed and the semen analysis was normal, it would be appropriate to wait for 6–12 months before seriously considering a myomectomy operation.

4. Depending on the size of the fibroids, three or four courses of gonadotrophin-releasing hormone (GnRH) injections at 4-weekly intervals may be given, to reduce the size of the fibroids prior to operating.

5. It may be necessary to change from myomectomy to a hysterectomy if there is excessive bleeding. This change of plan is rare and, since it may produce unnecessary anxiety, it is no longer stated in some units.

6. There are advantages and disadvantages. One may remove or exclude any subserous myomata but, of course, there is a risk of introducing infection. In this particular case the uterine cavity was not opened as the fibroids were predominantly subserous and easily shelled out of the uterus.

7. Approximately 40%.

8. Lesions with significant cytological atypia.

9. It is the patient's choice but, in the absence of a family history of ovarian cancer at 40 years, the ovaries, or at least one, should be conserved. The hyperplasia previously noted is not associated with the risk of carcinoma of the endometrium or ovary.

Case 217

1. **(a)** In this age group the mass is most likely to be a mature cystic teratoma (dermoid). These tumors form about 20% of all ovarian tumors and 90% are found in women who are of reproductive age. A high proportion of them, as in this case, are asymptomatic and it is an incidental finding.
   (b) Tumor markers that may be used are alphafetoprotein (AFP) and CA 125.

2. Yes, provided that the couple understand that there is a slight risk that the cyst might be malignant or undergo malignant change. In fact, a compromise was reached that the cyst would be removed towards the end of the second trimester of pregnancy. No specific discussion was made regarding corticosteroids or tocolytic agents.

3. The grade of the immature teratomas. An immature teratoma is a malignant tumor that implants upon the peritoneum and metastasizes to reach peritoneal tissues and para-aortic lymph nodes. Dissemination via the blood stream to the liver and lungs can occur. The prognosis of any case is determined by the degree and extent of immaturity. A widely used classification of immature teratoma is as follows:
   Grade 1 Minor foci of immature tissue. Rare mitotic activity.
   Grade 2 Moderate quantities of immature tissue with moderate mitotic activity.
   Grade 3 Large quantities of immature tissue.
   This grading system is of considerable prognostic value. In recent years, attention has been focused upon the amount of immature neuroepithelium present in the tumor as a prognostic guide (217b). The quantitation of the amount of this type of tissue aids prognosis. In about 10% of cases these tumors present with abdominal pain, of which torsion of the ovarian tumor is one cause.

4. The prognosis of immature solid teratoma of the ovary, until the last couple of decades, was extremely poor, the 5-year survival rate being less than 20%. Current therapeutic regimes are now holding out the promise of improved long-term survival, with sustained complete remissions being obtained in 90% of cases. Fertility is not usually impaired in survivors. The laparotomy on Mrs S was limited to inspection of the other ovary, which appeared to be normal, and there was no evidence of any free fluid. No peritoneal washings were taken. Either policy of action could be followed. However, because of the Grade 2 nature of the teratoma, with the patient's consent and desire for further pregnancies, a 6-month course of combination chemotherapy was considered the most appropriate policy and carried out in this case.

5. The differential diagnosis is: fibroids; ovarian cyst; ascites; and unusual bladder or bowel tumor. In a younger and premenopausal woman, pregnancy has to be considered.

6. The ultrasound scan, using Doppler, was very suggestive that this was an ovarian adenocarcinoma. There was no free fluid and the other ovary appeared quite normal. The kidneys and liver were normal.

7. **(a)** Arrange for a CT scan, repeat the CA 125 test, and decide whether or not chemotherapy should be given. A careful check on the family history did not indicate any deaths from breast, uterine, ovarian, or colonic cancer.
   (b) The prognosis for borderline tumors varies according to the type–mucinous (217e) or serous (217f). Our long-term follow-up indicates that 68% of women with borderline

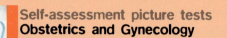

mucinous tumors survive 10 years, compared with 76% of the women with serous borderline tumors. It was also found that there was a higher proportion of the women with mucinous tumors who had late recurrences.

8.   HRT is not contraindicated, and a combined estrogen and progestogen preparation is preferred.

Case 218

1.   **(a)** A biopsy should be taken from the cancer for a histological diagnosis. The clinical staging would now be described as 1b1.
      (b) This staging would, of course, be changed to Stage III if hydronephrosis or hydroureter was revealed by an intravenous urogram (IVU) or other imaging techniques. In Ms A's case a CT scan revealed normal kidneys and ureters. Stage III carcinomas are treated by radiotherapy.

2.   Since 1994, FIGO Stage 1a is invasive cancer identified microscopically.
      Stage 1a1: measured stromal invasion no greater than 3 mm in depth and no wider than 7 mm.
      Stage 1a2: measured stromal invasion greater than 3 mm and no greater than 5 mm in depth and no wider than 7 mm.
      Larger lesions must be staged as 1b. Vascular space involvement, venous or lymphatic, does not alter the staging.
      Stage 1b1: lesions no greater than 4 cm.
      Stage 1b2: lesions greater than 4 cm.

3.   Every patient has the right to make an informed choice with regard to knowing the diagnosis and treatment options after being told of all the risks, actual and potential. The original plan had been referral for a Wertheim's hysterectomy 6–8 weeks after the first cone biopsy. This was deferred and a second cone biopsy carried out, with the acceptance by Ms B that it still might be appropriate to recommend a Wertheim's hysterectomy 6–8 weeks later. An MRI prior to the second cone biopsy in fact revealed no nodal involvement and only evidence of previous surgery to the cervix. The patient accepted the involved risks of a second cone biopsy operation and potential delay in treatment.

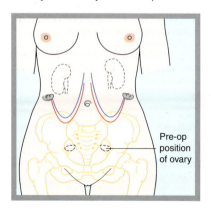

← **218g**

Pre-op position of ovary

4. Either (i) still recommend hysterectomy, conserve ovaries, and offer IVF, with surrogacy, after 5 years' follow-up or (ii) take 3-monthly smears routinely for 1–2 years. Arrange for repeat MRI in 6 months. On each occasion take ecto- and endocervical smears. If negative, try for pregnancy as soon as possible.

Pregnancy: Avoid pregnancy for 3 months then, if not successful in, say, 6–9 months, consider uterine insemination of the partner's sperm because of the loss of the major part of the vaginal cervix. If smears are positive opt for (i).

If not pregnant after 9–12 months consider IVF techniques and embryo replacement. Ms B was warned of the need for cervical suture if pregnancy occurred.

If a second MRI indicates that the nodes are enlarged, then either perform laparoscopy for biopsy/clearance of lymph nodes and subsequent management depending on histology, or remove them at the time of a Wertheim's hysterectomy.

5. The risk of ovarian metastases is less than 1% for women with squamous carcinoma and slightly higher for an adenocarcinoma. The ovaries should be placed as high as possible out of the pelvis and in a position possible for egg collection for IVF (see 218g). Marker metal clips should be applied to the pedicle for locating them, in order to avoid irradiating them if radiotherapy is used. The insistence by Ms C on a Pfannenstiel incision unfortunately did not allow either ovary to be placed high or lateral enough to be screened off from the subsequent external irradiation that was necessary.

6. Excessive hemorrhage and possible onset of abortion.

7. Yes, once the decision had been made to continue with the pregnancy. Early delivery (34–36 weeks) with the likelihood of survival of the child was appropriate. The blood vessels, particularly the veins, are bigger, but the surgical planes and ureters are more readily defined. A Cesarean section was carried out initially and the uterine incision closed after delivery of the child and the placenta. This was followed by a Wertheim's hysterectomy (ovaries conserved) and lymphadenectomy. The major risk is thromboembolism and appropriate preventative measures are essential in all cases.

8. If surgically treated cases subsequently require radiotherapy, infection can have an adverse effect on its effectiveness. Because there is, in general, a higher incidence of pelvic infection in women with carcinoma of the cervix, removal of the fallopian tubes is potentially beneficial. It also avoids the rare late complication of torsion or hydrosalpinx occurring.

9. **(a)** This is debatable with hindsight, hence the options for these later patients. The lesion in this case was multifocal and unlikely to have been completely excised, so radical surgery at that time was considered more appropriate, especially in light of the CT scan finding of an enlarged pelvic lymph node. A large cone biopsy might have been appropriate with careful follow-up.

(b) All four women will be followed up closely.

Ms A did require radiotherapy, despite at operation having negative pelvic and paracervical nodes. A CT scan 6 months later revealed enlarged nodes and she also later required chemotherapy. Ms A found it difficult to come to terms with the diagnosis and is unlikely to survive.

Ms B's problem might have been related to achieving a pregnancy but, in fact, she did conceive 6 months after the second cone biopsy and will be managed like Ms D.

Ms C has had recurrent disease despite radical radiotherapy. The long-term prognosis is, therefore, poor.

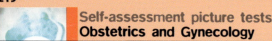
Ms D, in all probability, is cured and also has the child she desired because there was no residual disease found in the uterus nor the lymph nodes removed.

In summary, only two of the four are likely to be cured and they are the young women with the smaller, albeit multifocal, tumors, like Ms E. The young women with tumors of diameters 3 x 3 cm and 4 x 4 cm, respectively, already have been treated for recurrent disease and are not cured and are unlikely to survive.

Case 219

1. The common infection following the use of broad-spectrum antibiotics is monilial infection. However, with an episiotomy, staphylococci, streptococci, and coliforms are all common infecting bacteria.

2. A rectal examination is essential while getting the woman to contract her pelvic muscles at the same time in order to determine whether the sphincter ani and levator ani muscles are, or are not, deficient and intact. In this case it was evident that the episiotomy had extended into the external ani muscle and had not been recognized.

3. Bowel preparation preoperatively and intraoperative antibiotics would be appropriate.

4. Yes.

5. A diagram of an alternative type of graft is shown in 219f.

6. A third- or fourth-degree tear. Successful prolapse repair and possibly curative operation for stress incontinence.

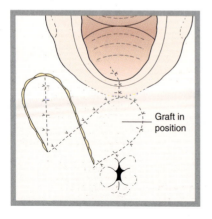

← **219f**

Graft in position

INDEX